Living
Through
Cancer

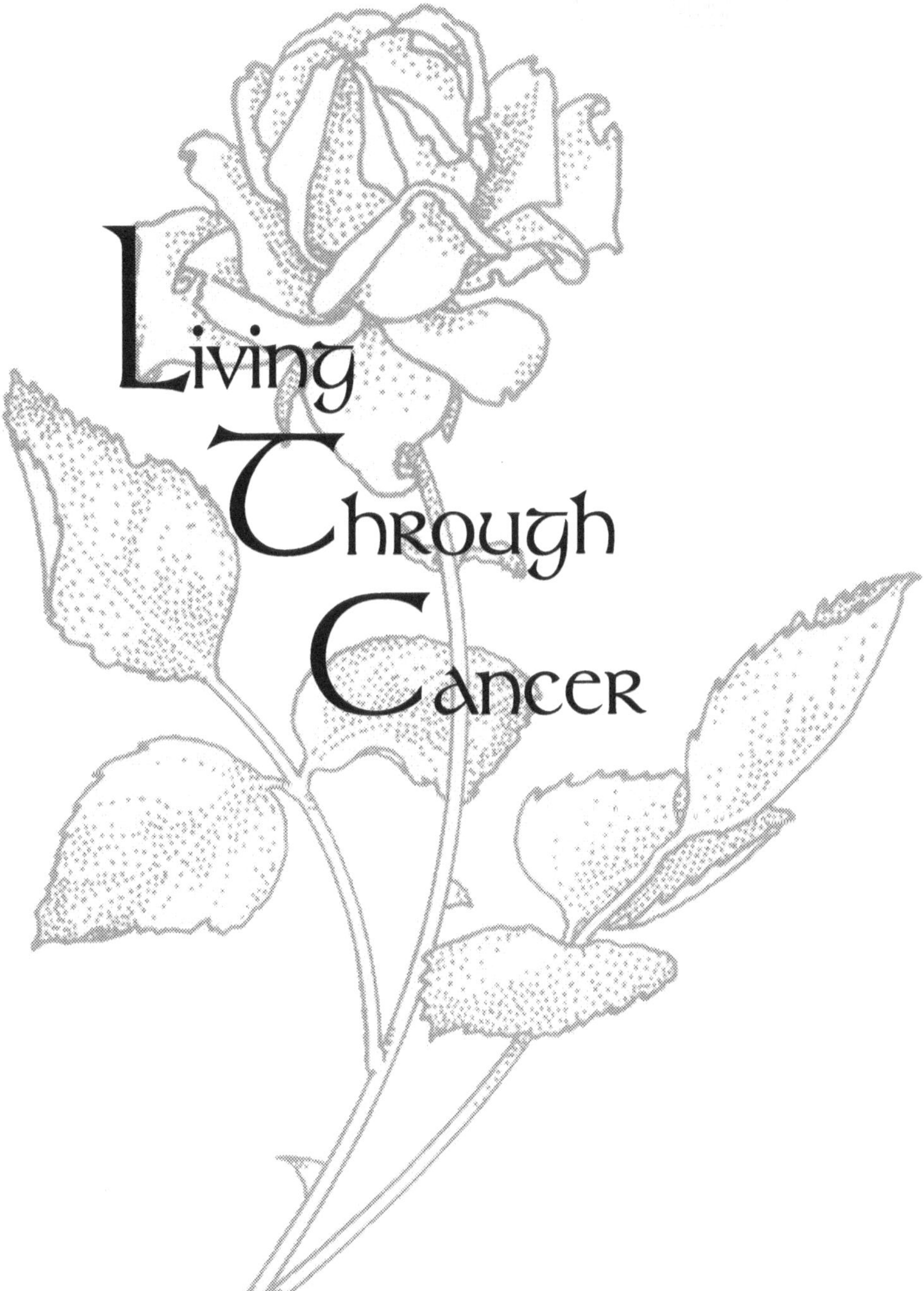

Testimonials

The author of *Living Through Cancer* was able to quickly establish an insightful analysis into the journey of dispair and hope and finally a resolution. The year Ken so lovingly cared for his beloved wife, Joan, was not a burden but a blessing. He showed the reader how to display love and adoration to the patient while never taking forgranted that he could 'do that tomorrow' for tomorrow may never come and all any of us have is today.

He was able to clearly show there are many rainbows after the storm.

Cancer can be a great blessing as you learn to 'live by faith, not sight'. When a cancer patient is at her weakest, the caregiver becomes strong. You learn not to take things forgranted and you find you have more friends than thought possible. But most importantly, one learns that 'God does provide a way'. From the moment one is diagnosed, they become victims but it is their chose to then become a survivor. Not to mention "Chemo" - just the word is enough to send a chill of fear down the spine but to worry is like sitting in a rocking chair - it gets you no where.

Now that I am ill and things look their worst, nothing is more inspiring to me than reading about how other people survived against the odds and cope with their situations. There are as many different ways to survive as there are patients and so we can learn something different from each other. Though we all face fear, panic and anxiety in our daily battle, we have our fair share of courage, fortitude and hope to win the war.

One of the more enlightening aspects I took away from reading the book is not to lose your sense of humor. I often tell my family not to worry because when I survive they would have worried for no reason and if the Lord finds reason otherwise, they will have time to cry for me later and that there is no need to do it twice. Attitude is everything in recovering from cancer. You gotta have 'tude if you expect to take a licking and come back ticking.

Thanks, Ken and Joan, for becoming the human voice of all cancer patients and their caregivers. How resolute you both have been in seeing this chapter in your life through, step by step and then so unselfishly sharing it with so many others.

—Dottie Judd

I would like to thank you, Ken for writing this book. It has prepared me for the recent news that my father, James Robert Banks, was diagnosed with lung cancer. Questions ran through my mind, what will my father go through? What kind of pain will he endure? I felt Lost and confused.

I remembered months prior to the news about my father, you would visit me and inform me of your wife's condition and her battle with cancer. I admired your strength and positive attitude.

I believe you are an angel that was sent to me to prepare for this time with your transcripts of your book and your encouraging words. My father is starting his radiation treatment and now I feel like I have a better understanding of what he'll have to endure. I have learned through your book that there is nothing like having family around with love and support when you are not feeling well. This is always, "Good Therapy."

The book has blessed me with encouragement and hope. I can only wish that you will have the opportunity to share your book with others who are experiencing cancer in their lives and to guide those who are feeling lost and confused.

—Diann McDonough

Must reading for a family with a cancer patient. An insightful day-by-day account of how a loving husband dealt with his wife's breast cancer and regimen of chemo and radiation therapy.

A beautiful and heartwarming story of a dedicated family coping with a major health crisis.

—Carol Cavanaugh

I knew that you guys were having a rough time of it, but after reading Ken's writings I truly understand what you have been going through.

The writing are truly "eye openers" and I'm sure would prove extremely helpful to anyone going through the same ordeal. Thank God for your strong love for each other, for your loving family's prayers and full support and for the prayers and support of your friends.

Joan and Ken, I know that with the strong faith that you both have in Him, that everything will be OK and you will both get back to a normal life.

—Doris White

Ken first approached me to ask if I would be willing to read his daily account of what he and Joan were living through. Of course I would do this! Little did I know it would unfold into what I term a FULL BLOWN LOVE STORY. Every few days he would bring a few more pages describing the challenges they both endured. They never lost sight of their goal. Joan was at times so weak. During a period like that Ken took up the slack. The heavy schedules they needed to follow just to get back and forth to the unbelievable but necessary number of appointment was taken in stride with no complaints. Ken was equally as diligent at seeing to it that Joan met her nail and hair appointments without fail. He knew how important they were to her. They took all the ups and downs together.

Ken will not take credit for all he did. He says Joan did the same for him years ago when he was seriously ill. Through it all these Lovers had a passion to beat the enemy together. And they remain optimistic that they have.

—Janet A. Child

Ken presents a wonderful true story of love and trust. After reading Ken's book, I just wanted to give him a hug for being the most caring, faithful and loving husband in the world. Each night I hated to leave Ken and Joan behind and longed to read more of their tale. I could hardly wait to resume their story of love and trust the next day. Ken made me feel the pain and joy alike as he recounted their journey out of the cruel shadow of cancer and chemo into a promise of renewed life. This is a poignant romantic tale of a lasting love.

—Rita Finn

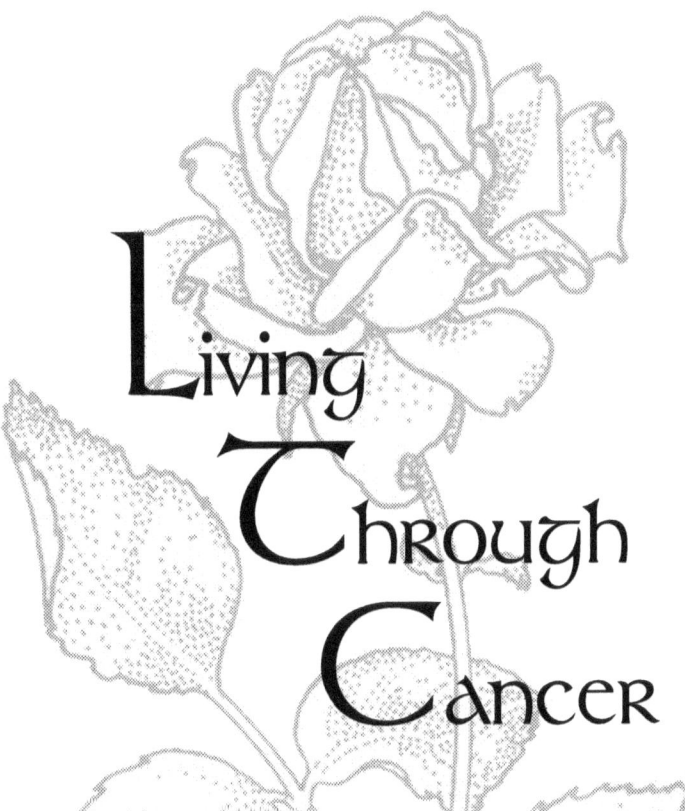

Living Through Cancer

A Story of Love and Caregiving

Kenneth R. Dickson

TRAFFORD

Note for Librarians: A cataloguing record for this book is available from Library and Archives Canada at www.collectionscanada.ca/amicus/index-e.html
ISBN 1-4120-5862-7

Printed on paper with minimum 30% recycled fibre. Trafford's print shop runs on "green energy" from solar, wind and other environmentally-friendly power sources.

TRAFFORD

Offices in Canada, USA, Ireland and UK
This book was published *on-demand* in cooperation with Trafford Publishing. On-demand publishing is a unique process and service of making a book available for retail sale to the public taking advantage of on-demand manufacturing and Internet marketing. On-demand publishing includes promotions, retail sales, manufacturing, order fulfilment, accounting and collecting royalties on behalf of the author.

Book sales for North America and international:
Trafford Publishing, 6E–2333 Government St.,
Victoria, BC v8t 4p4 CANADA
phone 250 383 6864 (toll-free 1 888 232 4444)
fax 250 383 6804; email to orders@trafford.com
Book sales in Europe:
Trafford Publishing (uk) Ltd., Enterprise House, Wistaston Road Business Centre,
Wistaston Road, Crewe, Cheshire cw2 7rp UNITED KINGDOM
phone 01270 251 396 (local rate 0845 230 9601)
facsimile 01270 254 983; orders.uk@trafford.com
Order online at:
trafford.com/05-0763

10 9 8 7 6 5 4 3 2

Dedication

To my God in heaven, without whom this book could not have been written. He is my strength in everything I do. To our wonderful family for all the love and support they give to Joan and me, every day of their lives. They dedicate their love and care to us always. To all our friends and loved ones who, in a very special way, gave their love and their many, many prayers. And to all those people who didn't even know us but took the time to pray for our Joan. God, you did give us a very special World.

Foreword

*T*he book you are about to read is about adversities, faith, and courage. Last but not least, love … all of which exists in everyone's life at one point or another.

How we survive the adversities that face us depends on the one freedom no one can ever take from us—our attitude and how we choose to deal with them.

Life doesn't stop because we feel bad, someone is hurt or sick or we lose someone dear to us in any way. The daily grind continues, and we must always face it.

My father—a man of great faith, strength, and compassion—wrote this book sharing the fears and uncertainties of my mother's illness while still living through everyday issues. Writing this book gave him a sense of purp9ose and helped him feel that his experiences could benefit others in similar situations.

My mother, diagnosed with breast cancer after always being diligent with her health and screenings, was devastated with fear of the unknown; but she turned around and showed more strength and courage than perhaps I ever could. She never questioned what needed to be done, she just pressed on even though she was scared and chemically weakened. Her love for life and family outweighed it all.

Their life together began in love and faith. Their family was born out of love and faith. Their courage and strength held together by that love and faith. They faced adversities daily-some cancer related and some not. Together they fought the toughest battle of their lives.

Doreen

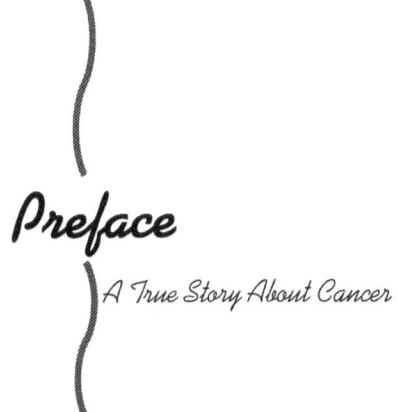

Preface

A True Story About Cancer

I t all began, the second week in March of 2003, with a mammogram.

My wife, Joan, had a history of non-cancerous cysts and calcium
deposits. In 1996, she had a partial mastectomy proving to be non-
cancerous. These uncertain cysts along with the fact that Joan's mother
had cancer, concluding in a full mastectomy, led the doctor to the wise
decision to schedule Joan every six months for a mammogram. Little did
we know, how life could change in six months time.

Doctor Vopal examined carefully Joan's mammography and noticed a
concernable spot. The spot was near the surface, which was promising, but
a biopsy was ordered for safety sake. The needle plunged into my wife's soft
tissue like a heat-seeking missile and quickly located the dubious area.

The days between the biopsy and the next meeting with the doctor drug
on with our fears getting the best of us. We believe that God is in control
and will help those who help themselves. Meaning if you are wise in
preventative medicine for your body, things should be OK. God gave us
what we have and it is up to us to take care of what He has bestowed upon
us. We strive to be responsible and caring children for all the beautiful
astonishing wonders God has given us.

The day arrived for our appointed Doctor's visit, the day that will forever
be stamped across my heart - March 31, 2003. Dr. Vopal carefully but
skillfully laid out the bad news first. Joan had a tumor in the breast right
under the partial mastectomy area. Then we heard the "C" word and life
as we had known it passed before our eyes. Joan had a cancerous tumor

and it would need to be removed. We felt as if Novocain had been shot into our veins. We were numb with shock. Almost too numb to absorb the coming good news.

Doctor Vopal continued on telling us that he felt this situation was fixable between the surgery, chemotherapy and radiation therapy. Fixable - what a magnificent word!

We had fourteen days to fill between the day of reckoning and the day of the operation which was scheduled for April 14. One of the first tasks was to alert our children to these new developments. It is always very difficult for children of any age to cope well when they hear a parent is threatened with disease. Our children were active in questions and we discussed everything from second opinions to the quality of doctors. We all agreed that we were in the best caring hands possible with Doctor Vopal. You can't do better than having a doctor that is known to be the best in their field. Before we knew it the operation day was upon us.

The operation would take place in Martin Memorial Hospital located in Stuart, Florida and my wife, now a victim of cancer, would be rolled away from my grasping hands for this surgery at six in the morning on that April day. We knew the chemo would be starting soon after the operation. The first treatment had already been scheduled for April 30. Doctor Iannotti would be in charge of the chemo program and we would soon be meeting Doctor Griffis to learn about the radiation program.

Our son Ken and our daughters Kim and Diane hovered over us with their concern, support and tender love. Our daughter Doreen could not be there which was emotionally devastating to her. Her husband was away and her responsibility was to her own children at home. Some how we knew she too was hovering over us along with the ones that were physically there.

It is amazing how operations are now adays. After we knew the operation was successful, we stayed for Joan to recuperate and then we scooted home as if all this had been a blur; yet, we knew we were facing the dreaded chemo.

A few days passed and Joan was feeling better. If she was in a lot of pain, she did her best to not show it. It is hard for a man to see the ones he is supposed to protect and care for suffer any kind of emotional or physical pain. You want to make it all go away and for life to be enemy free. I knew Joan had been dealt a formidable opponent but she faced this with a commitment to win. I am a very proud husband.

Ken Dickson

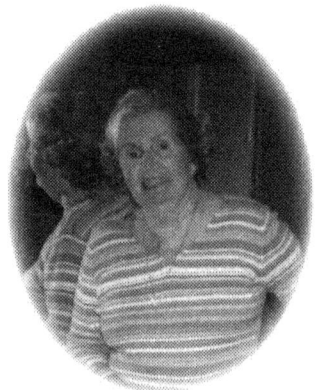

The Joan A. Dickson Story

These notes were taken directly from my diary with very little editing. I wanted the full impact of what I was feeling to be open and honest without filtering.

My hope and goal is by sharing my daily writings, it will help others.

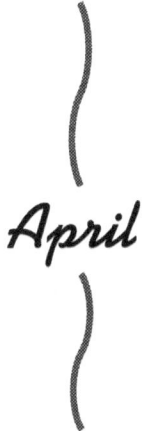

April

April 14, 2003

Remove Tumor from left breast and 34 nodes under left arm of which one node had a microscopic amount of cancer in it. Operation was a one day surgery procedure. Joan was home that night.

April 17, 2003

Joan had a follow up appointment with doctor Vopal. Everything OK.

April 24, 2003 and April 29, 2003

Joan had follow up appointments with Dr. Vopal. At this time doctor Vopal suggested we follow up with Doctor Iannotti for chemo treatment. We were also to follow up with Dr. Griffis for radiology treatment.

April 30, 2003

Joan had first appointment with Doctor Iannotti in Fort Pierce FL. We talked about the operation along with the follow up procedure. Doctor Iannotti suggested a program of chemo once a month for three months, radiation every day for six weeks Monday through Friday. After that, we would be back to three more shots of chemo over the next three months. He also suggested that Joan have a PET test [a new procedure]. The pet test is to find out if there is any more cancer elsewhere. The Doctor's all agreed this test is not conclusive but gives a general idea of where to look if there were any indications of cancer. We said we would have the test. The Doctor's nurse made an appointment for the test on May 13, 2003.

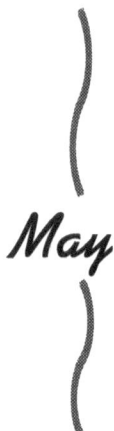

May

May 13, 2003

Joan had the PET test at the Port St. Lucie Radiology Unit. It took the better part of the afternoon to do this. We called the Doctor's office on the next day and were told to call back on Friday the 16th.

May 17, 2003

Spoke with Doctor Iannotti. He wanted Joan to have a scan under her left arm, the same area where her operation had been. He said Joan was to have stage two chemo, not stage one, after looking at the results of the PET scan. [The operation under the arm was where the nodes were taken out.] The chemo was to be a stronger amount and to be over four months instead of six months. This would change the schedule to four months of chemo instead of six months, [one shot a month]. Radiation would start after the chemo was finished. Radiation would be for about six weeks - every day except Saturday and Sunday.

May 19, 2003

Doctor Iannotti wanted Joan to have a heart scan. An under arm scan was performed and the results given to Doctor Iannotti.

May 27, 2003

Joan had heart scan done - results given to Doctor Iannotti. [Both under arm and heart scans were done at the Port St Lucie Radiation Bldg.]

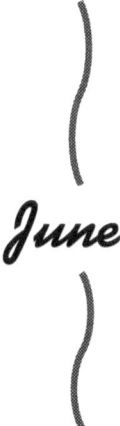

June

June 2, 2003

We called Doctor Iannotti for results of the two scans. The under arm scan did not change anything. The heart scan showed her heart to be OK. An appointment was then made for Friday, June 6th with Doctor Iannotti in his Stuart office at 3:30 PM to discuss everything to date and to make arrangements to have Doctor Vopal insert the "port" so we can start the chemo sessions.

June 6, 2003

Arrangements were made with Doctor Vopal's office to have the operation for the "port" to be put in on June 13th [Friday]. We than made an appointment to start the Chemo at 10:30 A.M., the same day with Doctor Iannotti.

June 13, 2003

We arrived at the Martin Memorial Surgery Center at 6:15 to have the operation for the Port to be inserted into Joan's right side of the upper part of her chest. [The Port is used to eliminate being stuck with needles and IV's]. Everything went OK and after Joan rested we wheeled her in her wheel chair to Doctor Iannotti's office for Joan's first Chemo procedure at 10:30 A.M. The procedure took [with waiting time] about two hours. Things went well and we were on our way home about 12:30 or 1:00 P.M. After arriving home we were both exhausted and fell sound asleep for at least two to three hours. Joan didn't have any problems that night except for a small amount of nausea.

June 14 & 15, 2003

Joan seemed to be fine, outside of being tired and some feelings of nausea. We even went to the mall for a short while. Did OK

June 16 & 17, 2003

Joan woke up on the 16th [Monday] not feeling too well– she ached and had feelings of nausea all day. She could not eat well all day and had to skip dinner. On the 17th Joan had a good breakfast and had lunch about 2:30 P.M. We will see how the rest of the day goes. Joan is still pretty tired and achy but better then the 16th - Ooops spoke too soon. Joan was thinking of eating something since she did not want to eat dinner. Just the thought of eating for some reason made her throw up. It was the first time she threw up since she had Chemo on the 13th of June.

June 18, 2003

After Joan threw up last night, she rested and fell asleep about 11:30 PM until 8:00 A.M. this morning. So far today she has not been sick but has been very, very tired. She slept most of the morning until 1:30 p.m. We are thinking about lunch but nothing sounds good to Joan. [We will figure it out.] Had lunch and supper and Joan rested. She was still very tired and had slight feeling of nausea at the end of the day.

June 19, 2003

Joan had appointment with Doctor Vopal to remove bandage from the port operation. Everything was OK. Doctor Vopal put on another small bandage and told us to use vitamin E on the incision when the bandage falls off. We are to see Doctor Vopal on July 15th at 2:15 PM for a follow up appointment. The rest of the day seemed to go a little better; no throwing up but still a little nausea. It was our Daughter Kim's 40th Birthday and we were to go to her house for Birthday cake, but neither of us was feeling up to it.

June 20, 2003

Joan had appointment with Doctor Iannotti for a blood test at 2:00 PM. The blood count seemed to be a little low but OK. Joan told Doctor Iannotti about throwing up and her nausea feeling. Doctor Iannotti told

Joan that he would change the medicine for nausea to something stronger if it continues. He also gave Joan samples of Zoloft to relax her.

June 21 & 22, 2003

Joan seems to be much better, not to much nausea and no throwing up, although she is still very tired. No Doctor appointments for awhile. No hair loss yet.

June 23, 2003

Today Joan got up about 10:00 AM. She felt no nausea and she was feeling a little better. She had a good breakfast and lunch but no appetite for supper. About 3:00 PM we went to the store to buy some cards and a few other things we needed. After we came home Joan fell apart and became very tired. We called it a day and just took it easy until bed time.

June 24, 2003 Tuesday - Joan feels pretty good today as far as having an upset stomach. No Nausea. Joan's main problem now is that she is tired most of the time and has a lot of pain in her legs from the knees down to her ankles. The pain in her legs is not related to her cancer problem. Today we went to the mall for about one hour to return a shirt and have lunch. Joan seemed to handle the outing well. The rest of the day was spent at home taking it easy until bed time.

June 25, 2003

Joan and I got up early today, 7:30 AM. New chairs for the bedroom are arriving this morning. Joan feels pretty good; no nausea and legs not hurting as much so far. Joan is not as tired today so will keep her nail appointment this afternoon. Nails were done and supper out of the way. Time to put the t/v on and relax again. This was a pretty good day.

June 26, 2003

We got up about 8:30 AM. Today Joan has an appointment with Neil, her hair stylist. Kim and Sierra came for lunch today. We had a great time playing with Sierra. After Kim and Sierra left we went for Joan's hair appointment. She is now showing some hair loss, not a lot but some is showing up on the comb. Also Neil, Joan's hairdresser, noticed it. After supper we will watch t/v till bed time.

June 27, 2003

We got up about 11: 30 - must have been real tired. Joan feels pretty good as far as nausea goes. Hair loss is increasing and we both feel depressed about it. We had a long talk about the hair loss and decided there was nothing we can do about it, so guess we will just have to learn to live with it. After all it is just until the chemo is over and then Joan will get all her hair back. Every thing else seems to be going OK.

June 28, 2003

Everything seems to be OK. No nausea but a lot of hair loss. We went to the mall to buy hats for Joan, had a good time picking them out. On our way home we stopped for dinner. That was all for today.

June 29, 2003

About the same as Saturday except no mall. More hair loss. Most of the hair loss is in the back of the head. Joan's appetite seems to be a little better - not much but a little better.

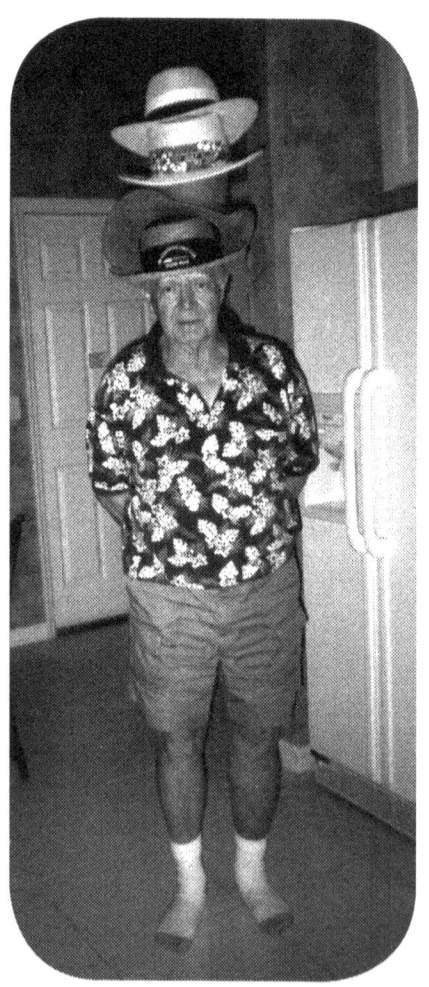

June 30, 2003

Nothing scheduled today and we took it easy all day. Hair loss is increasing, front of her head still not too bad but the back of her head - almost no hair left.

Voice of the Children

What was your first reaction to hearing the news your mother had cancer?

When I first found out about my mom's cancer I was not surprised because my Grandmother (her mother) had it. I was very nervous for her because I knew it would be a difficult time. I knew my dad would be very supportive and strong but I wished I lived closer so I could be of more help. *Diane*

My first reaction was a combination of mis-belief and realization that this was bound to happen sooner or later. My mother's mother had breast cancer and as we know it can be hereditary. I am just thankful that my mother was also aware that she needed to keep on top of her checkups and never miss her mammograms. We were also very fortunate that this was caught at an early stage. I thank God that it was a curable cancer. My parents have definitely had their share of health problems and I just couldn't believe that there was yet another obstacle that they had to endure. I do believe that they concurred it together with their love for each other and strength. *Kim*

I was surprised because I know how diligent my mother was in having regular check ups for breast cancer. Her mom had cancer so I knew she frequently had herself checked out. Of course, I was also very concerned not knowing how severe her diagnosis was. *Ken*

My first reaction surprisingly was not a surprise to me. I was very upset but knew my mom was a high risk to begin with. She had had several biopsies performed in the past and her mom had breast cancer at 64. Her mom survived breast cancer and died at 84 years old from unrelated circumstances. I was confident they had found my mom,s early enough to get it under control. None of us thought including the doctors that it was not as bad as it was until they actually got in there. Now the journey begins. *Doreen*

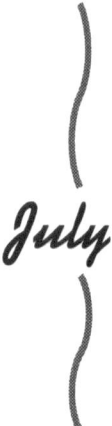

July

July 1, 2003

Ken had Doctor's appointment with Doctor Barrett in the morning. Joan had Doctor's appointment with Doctor Kass regarding her legs. Joan's legs seem to be improving. Doctor Kass increased the strength of the medicine [Neurontin] to 200 mgs. Doctor Kass feels Joan has some improvement in her walking and the pain is not as much as it was. Hair loss still increasing. Joan seems less tired today and was wearing the turban and one of the hats for a few hours.

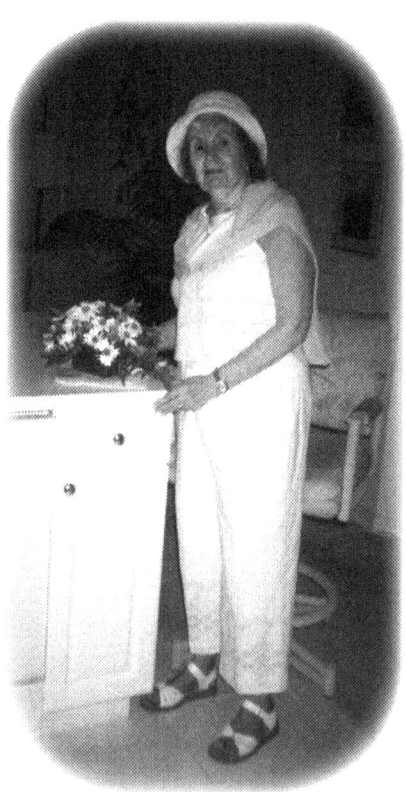

July 2, 2003

Today we went to a retirement party at a neighbor's house. It started at 3:00 PM and ended at 6:00 PM. Joan had a good time, she enjoyed talking to a lot of people that she has not seen for a long time. Joan wore a blue outfit o with a blue hat that we bought at the mall; she looked very nice. I think it did her good to get out. All in all it was a good day.

July 3, 2003

A quiet day at home, no Doctor's or appointments to keep. Joan has lost a lot of her hair and still looks as good as the gal I married. No ill effects from the chemo today.

July 4, 2003

Another quite day at home. Joan felt a little nauseous today not sure why, but we thought it better that we took it easy. We watched the Macy's Fireworks and called it a day.

July 5, 2003

Joan felt better today, no nausea. We did some things at home and watched tennis and golf all afternoon. Went out for dinner at a new restaurant and then came home. Guess what? We took it easy and then went to bed. Boy, are we getting rested.

July 6, 2003

Joan feeling pretty good today, no nausea but almost out of hair. Joan still very tired, falls asleep very easily, Chemo will make you very tired [so the doctor said]. It was a very nice day out today, about 95 degrees but not too humid, so I worked out side for a bit. All in all a good day [P.S. - Joan was a little depressed today, too much on her mind thinking about what is going on with her.]

July 7&8, 2003

Monday not much going on today. Joan feels achy all over but nothing really wrong. Tuesday was about the same as Monday. Joan has been thinking about going to chemo on Friday, the 11th and I guess it makes her a little nervous. This will be her second chemo procedure and she will only have two more to go. In October she will start her radiation program which should take about four to six weeks. The radiation treatments are five [5] days a week. After the radiation we should be able to get back to normal [WE HOPE].

July 9 & 10, 2003

Wednesday, not much going on today either, except for Joan's nail appointment. Joan put on her wig for the first time going out, she wore it to the nail salon and they thought she looked great, she will feel much better next time she wears it I'm sure. Thursday, Joan felt pretty good, not as tired as she has been feeling. We did much of nothing except I got a haircut and took my granddaughter to soccer practice. Kim came over with Sierra to pick up Sammy, which is always a delight. We watched T/V and went to bed.

July 11 & 12, 2003

Friday we got up at 8:30 AM. so we would be ready for Joan's appointment for her Chemo. We had a good breakfast and just took it easy until it was time to leave. No problems – we talked to Doctor Iannotti before the treatment. Joan needed two prescriptions and wanted to have the doctor look at her tongue, to see if it was any better. The Doctor said she should continue with the medication until it was all cleared up. After Joan's treatment we went to get something to eat and than went home. No apparent effects from the shot as of 9:00 PM tonight. [Will see how tomorrow goes.] P.S. – The tongue has nothing to do with the cancer problem, it is an infection of the tongue called Rush which the Doctor is also treating. We are glad the day is over.

Saturday - Joan felt pretty good today. No nausea as yet, just very tired. Joan rested all day, maybe she will feel like doing something on Sunday. PPS - Joan did not tell me until now that she has had a headache [dull one] since the chemo shot, she also had the runs and is very red in the face [looks very flush in the face].

July 13, 2003

Got up about 9: 00 AM. , had breakfast, read the paper and got ready to, guess what, you got it, we are going to spend another day relaxing. Joan seems to be feeling pretty good, she is still very tired but no feeling of nausea as yet. Joan takes the nausea pills when she is supposed to. I guess it works if you do it right. Joan has no appetite, she can't pick out anything that she wants to eat. Nothing appeals to her [EXCEPT ICE CREAM SODAS]

Oops - I guess I spoke too soon, about 10: 00 PM Joan looks not to good, she feels very nauseous and looks kind of pale, hopefully it will pass. This is two days after her chemo shot, the same time interval as the first time she had her shot. Joan did not throw up and hopefully she won't. It is now 12:30 AM and it looks like she has fallen asleep, maybe the nauseous feeling has left.

July 14, 2003

Joan had a good night sleep considering how she felt last night. Today seems to be about the same as last night before Joan fell asleep. She has been nauseous all day, along with an aching body and being super tired. It has not been a good day. Hope Joan can get to sleep tonight like she did last night. She had a good breakfast this morning [It was more like lunch]. We ate breakfast at 12:00 PM . As far as eating goes the rest of the day it has not been to nutritional and she ate very little. I guess when you feel nauseous you do not feel like eating anything. Hope tomorrow will be better.

July 15, 2003

Well today is here and it did not change from yesterday. Joan is still nauseous and very tired along with aching all over. Joan went through the day and still does not have a feeling for eating anything. Today she had breakfast, which she seems to tolerate. But the rest of the day was like yesterday, she did not want to eat outside of some fruit and part of a sandwich - no supper. Joan did throw up tonight but nothing really came up. I guess it was what they call the dry heaves. After Joan threw up she felt a little better or at least it seemed like she felt better. She even looked better. Guess we will have to see how things go through the night. PS - Joan has been burping a lot the last few days. It must be a sign of something but who knows what. Guess it will be a question for the Doctor.

July 16, 2003

Today Joan woke up feeling better. She only threw up the one time last night, which is an improvement from last month when she became ill from the chemo shot. It seems that after Joan gets her chemo shot, it does not bother her for about one to two days then, whammo, it hits her like a ton of bricks. She gets nauseous, throws up and basically feels like she was run over by a truck. She must feel better; she asked me to pick up some candy she likes. She did not eat it yet but at least she felt good enough to want me to get it for her. Joan looked better today than she has in the past few days. Joan's hair has not been falling out like it was. I guess it could be that there isn't anything up there to come out any more. She has some strands of hair at the edges of her head, and that's about it. She still looks good to me with or without the hair. Joan's diet today consisted of Taylor ham on a roll [which is her favorite] and orange juice. For lunch she had peanut butter on seven saltines and a small glass of Diet Coke. Supper consisted of chicken noodle soup, saltine crackers and a glass of water. Tomorrow I'm sure she will want something more solid. At least I hope so. It is now time to watch some T/V and go to bed.

July 17, 2003

Today was a nothing day, by that I mean we stayed at home and did exactly what ever we wanted to do. Joan felt pretty good – no nausea feelings and not too much aching with the body. Joan's hair I think is about done falling out. There is hardly any hair left. Joan doesn't look too bad with out hair.

She has a nicely shaped head, at least I think so. I sometimes seem to make light of what is going on with us, [if I didn't I think we would be in big trouble]. Joan has her bad moments but is a real trooper handling it. I'm proud of her and the way she is copping. Cancer and the treatment getting rid of it sucks, please excuse the language but it really does suck. I guess what makes it tolerable is that the Doctor's say they got it all and Joan will be OK when the treatment is all over. We pray to God that they are right and I'm sure that they are. We have about three and one half months to go with the treatment and about six months of Joan getting her hair back. Then we will feel back to normal. I do run on so I think I will say goodnight. "Goodnight".

July 18, 2003

Today Joan has an appointment to have her blood checked. We will have to go to Stuart to the cancer center to do so. Our appointment is at three PM and it should not take more than a half hour to draw the blood and to have the lab give us a report on how the red and white cells are behaving. The report was not too bad; both the red and the white cells were low but not to a dangerous point.

Joan is on the fence with being anemic, but that to can be corrected. After we left the center we decided to go to a new store we heard about to buy some fruit. The trip was worth it. The fruit was really good. We had supper and are now ready for a short night of T/V and then to bed. 'Goodnight ". PS - Joan handled the day OK.

July 19, 2003

We woke up about 8:30 AM. Luise was coming to finish up the yard work. It is a weekend so there is no procedures for Joan meaning we can do what ever we want. I had a bad morning,[felt light headed most of the morning.] Joan was very worried and was taking care of me as best she could. I felt better in the afternoon, about 2:00 PM and could see the relief on Joan's face right away. I guess we just worry about each other to much. Must be Love. We watched golf off and on all day. The night was guess what ? You got it –T/V and bed. "Goodnight "

PS: Joan felt pretty good today - no nausea or aching but still tired.

July 20, 2003

Today is going to be a very good day, our daughter Diane and our grand-daughter Kerri and grandson AJ will be here for a week visit. This is what I call real good therapy. Joan feels pretty good today, no nausea or aching to speak of. Her hair has stabilized, sort of. It seems to be growing but that must be an allusion, or something wrong with my eyes. There is nothing like having family around when you do not feel good. Our other daughter Doreen will be here next month for a visit with us. Kim, our daughter that lives five minutes from us is by our side every day. Believe it or not, this is the best medicine that any one could prescribe. Ken, our son, and his family were here in June and they are in touch with us on a weekly basis. We have had so much support from our family and close friends, that we didn't feel a need for a support group. However, it sure is a good feeling knowing that the support groups are just a phone call away. There are a lot of good people on this Earth of ours, more than a lot of people think. The not so good people are in the minority but for some reason seem to be in the limelight more. Our kids arrived and settled in for a while, so I guess we'll call it a day.

July 21, 2003

Today we got up about 10:00 AM. We must have been tired and had a hard time just getting out of bed. We did not have anything on our sched-ule so we just hung out for the day. Joan was feeling pretty good so we made dinner reservations for five [Joan –Diane – Kerri – AJ and myself] at the Manor. The Manor is a very nice restaurant in the PGA Reserve. We had a very nice time and Joan handled it well. After dinner we left for home and called it a day, or so we thought. No sooner we got into bed and all hell broke out. Yep, Joan got sick and it took us until 5:00 in the morning until she felt somewhat better. I don't think we got more than one or two hours sleep all night. We don't think it was what she ate. Joan said it was the same feeling that she gets after she gets her chemo shot.

Joan had stopped taking the medicine to stop the nausea the day before, just like she did last month when the nauseous feeling left and she felt OK. We don't know why she got so sick but it sure was a tough night. We will have to ask the Doctor if she should continue on the medicine for nausea even after she feels better. I guess there is no rhyme or reason to this whole procedure, you just have to roll with it.

July 22, 2003

After getting almost no sleep last night we did absolutely nothing at all today. Joan did not feel or get nauseous or sick at all today. Needles to say she went back on the nausea medicine and will stay on it until we hear from the Doctor. Diane and AJ came over in the afternoon to see how Joan was. They stayed for supper and then went back to the condo early so Joan and I could get to bed early. I guess we had better stay on our guard and not try to rush the healing process, this is not something to fool with or to try and second guess it. Goodnight see you all tomorrow.

July 23, 2003

Had a good nights sleep. We woke up about 10:30 AM. . We had breakfast and got dressed for the day. Joan has an appointment to have her nails done and she does not want to miss that. Since she does not go to Neil for her hair she makes certain that she makes her nail appointments. Joan feels pretty good today, no nausea to speak of. Joan is still very tired and will probably be so until chemo is over with. Joan's hair has still stopped coming out, it looks like she is as bald as she is going to be. She still looks pretty good to me. Joan is putting on the wigs more often and is getting the hang of doing it. The wigs really look very nice, not as good as her own hair but they do look very nice on her. It looks like chemo knocks you out when you first get the shot and then for about ten days after. Except for being very tired she acts almost normal. I must say that Joan seems to day dream a lot. I'm sure she does not even know it. She seems to look into space and is miles away, I don't ever remember her doing that before. I guess she has a lot of thinking to do, or maybe she is simply tired. Well the kids stopped in to visit, so we will sign off for the night. See you tomorrow. Goodnight.

July 24, 2003

Last night Joan told me that she was having trouble when she urinates. She said it burned and was very uncomfortable. Joan has had trouble in this department before and it always ended up being a urinary infection.. With the chemo she is going through, her resistance towards infections is low, so we decided to call the Doctor . Joan called Doctor Ionnatti and was told to come to his office in Stuart at 3:00 PM today. After being tested Joan was told she did have a urinary infection and was given antibiotics for it. Hopefully it will take care of the infection quickly and make Joan feel better. She has enough to cope with and does not need anything else to bother her. I think we both have had it, and that it is time we started to get our act together and make ourselves think more positive about what is going on in our lives. It might take awhile to change things for a more positive outlook, so we had better start now. We have a lot of things to do, and a lot of time left to do them. We just have to put ourselves in the right mode and start having some fun, the health problems might take awhile to get straightened out but here is no reason why our mental outlook can't start improving now.

July 25, 2003

Nothing on the agenda this morning so we just took our time doing whatever. Joan wanted to wash her hair, so that's what we did. It didn't take long, I wonder why. All I know is that Joan felt better doing it. I washed and she dried. What a combo. In the afternoon Joan and I went to the mall with Diane –Kim –and Kerri. Kim drove so it was a very easy trip for me. Joan seems to feel better in regards to the infection she has. I think the antibiotic is doing its job. Also, Joan does not have any nausea today and that is a plus. I still think Joan's hair is growing. She thinks I'm out of my mind, but it sure looks like it to me. On that note I think we'll say goodnight.

PS- I think that we can cope with everything as long as we are doing it together. [there is no doubt about it, we are doing it together.]

July 26, 2003

After we awoke we had breakfast and got ready for another day. Most of the morning was spent on the phone talking to Marcia, Madiline, and our kids. Joan feels OK today except for being real tired. Diane wanted us to go to the beach, but neither Joan nor I had the energy. Instead, we caught up on a few things around the house that we have neglected with Diane Kerri and AJ visiting. Our children have been good about giving Joan the support that she needs. They visit us or call us on a daily basis. Diane Kerri and AJ are leaving tomorrow for NJ. It's going to be strange not having them around. Tonight we are all going out to dinner since it is their last night here. Joan is resting up this afternoon so she will have enough pep tonight. I will let you know how the night went when I talk to you tomorrow.

July 27, 2003

Last night was a real good night. We went to RJ Gators for dinner and we had a great time. AJ Gators is a restaurant that is kid orientated. It has games, music to dance to and the food is very good. The food is also kid orientated. We arrived at the restaurant at 7:00 PM and didn't leave until almost 10:00 PM . The kids were having a great time in the game room and it gave us oldies a chance to visit and have a conversation un-interrupted. Today our daughter Diane and our grandchildren Kerri and AJ left for NJ. The limo was picking them up at 9:00 AM. at our house so they had to be here at 8:00 AM for breakfast, and to say goodbye. We hated to see them go but hopefully it won't be to long until we see them all again. While they were here, it gave Joan just what she needed, time to get her mind off what she is going through. She put on one of her new wigs, and dressed up for the occasion. She looked real good and she had a real good time. When Joan is happy and smiling she is really beautiful inside and out. The rest of the day was spent taken it easy and having a little nap. Joan felt pretty good, still no nausea and tires easily. Joan's infection seems to be doing OK. She will stay on the medicine until it is all gone, then will be tested again with a blood test to make sure It is all better. We are now tired and headed for bed.

July 28, 2003

Today I'm sure will be a very quite day, and a little sad day, seeing that Diane and Kids are not here. We always feel sad for a few days after family goes back to NJ. I don't know whether it is because we didn't go with them or just because they're gone. Joan says she feels a little shaky today. Her walking is not to steady and very, very, very slow. We went to the store to get some fruit, and it took us forever, or so it seemed. Other than feeling slow and shaky, Joan has a little nausea and is very tired. We will eat supper and do as little as possible for the rest of the day.

P.S. Another thing that has us feeling sad is the news about Bob Hope passing away. He sure was a big part of everyone's life and will be missed very much. We love you BOB.

July 29, 2003

Today, Joan has an appointment with Doctor Vopal in Stuart, for a check up on how everything is going. Our appointment is at 2:15 PM , so we have to go at 1:30 PM to be there on time. It really doesn't matter because we wait in the office for at least one half hour before they call you into the exam room, and sometimes you wait another half hour before the Doctor gets into the exam room to see you. The good part about waiting is, the Doctor is not in a rush when he is with you and that is a very good thing. He really explains what is going on and will not leave you until you know and understand what he tells you. If you have questions, fire away and he is sure to answer all you have to ask. Today he told us that everything is going just fine. He did a hands-on exam on Joan and said every thing seems to be OK and that he would see Joan again in six months after the chemo and radiation is all done. To us that was a good sign. At least it is going in the right direction for a change. After the visit we went directly home. We were going to stop at the mall to get one of Joan's wigs fixed but Joan and I were both too tired to do so. We ordered Chinese for supper and took it very easy the rest of the night. See you tomorrow. Goodnight.

July 30, 2003

Hi! Another day about to start. No Doctor's or appointments to keep, just another quite day for us to handle. I sometimes wonder, is it better to be busy with appointments, Doctor's or other s, or is it better just to stay at home and rest? I'd really like to go to the beach or golf or do something of interest and I'm sure Joan would also. Oh well, we only have three more months to go. The main thing is to get Joan healthy again so we can live our lives. Sometimes I guess we get a little down and bored with the taking it easy and resting. Not having any visitors today, allowed us to get a lot of rest. Joan slept a lot and I worked on my computer and some paper work that needed to be done. I forgot I did bring the car in for service this morning. How did I ever forget that? I was gone for at least 20 minutes! We really do OK and get along with each other very well. Must be that we are used to each other and I guess we do like each other [must be love.] P.S. Joan was a little nauseated today. It came out of no where, but didn't last long.

July 31, 2003

Joan is very tired today and a little nauseous. She did not get sick but just didn't feel right. I, too, was very tired today. Joan has been taking her nausea pills for the last couple of days which is why she doesn't throw up. The day I'm sure will just be a take it easy day. We do have a man coming to clean the driveway at 3:30 PM and I'm sure that will end the day for us. Supper and to bed.

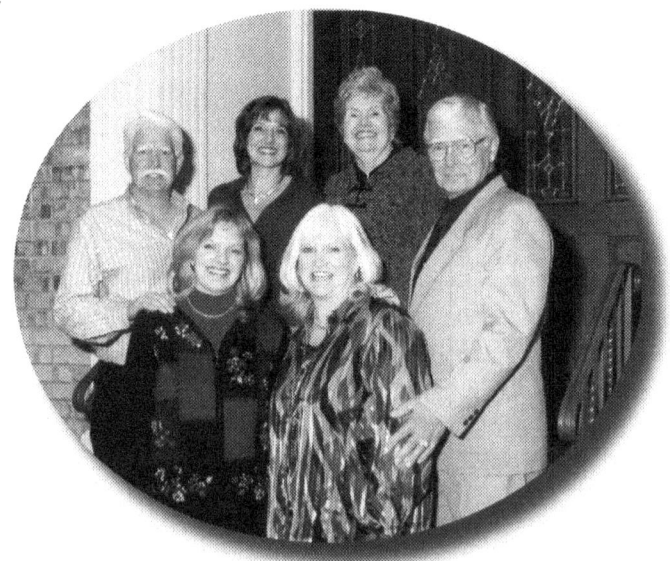

Voice of the Children

How did you feel you should participate in showing support for your mom and dad?

Because I lived so far away I knew I could only be supportive over the phone and with an occasional visit. It was very difficult for me when times were tough not to just jump on a plane. I wanted so much to just be able to give them both a hug. I was there during my mom's operation. After that I called almost every day. A lot of times she was too weak to talk to so I just spoke with my dad. She surprised me how strong she was through even the most difficult times. She always had a positive outlook. I was so proud of her. *Diane*

I tried to help as much as possible. Being a mother of four, as my mother knows, is very demanding. We live in the same town so I could keep an eye on them, although I couldn't get there everyday. If they really needed me I wasn't very far. Sometimes all they needed was a visit from their grandchildren to get their minds off of their problems. *Kim*

I wanted to be in Florida with them throughout the whole ordeal. Unfortunately, I knew that I could not, so I wanted to make sure I could at least be there for the surgery. I was able to spend a couple days with them after the surgery and than I knew that my sister, Kim, who lives near my parents, would be there to help them with whatever they needed. *Ken*

The hardest thing about being so far away from someone you love who is ill is you can,t get to them fast enough my parents live in Port Saint Lucie and I live in New Jersey. My arms are just not long enough and hugs were definitely needed. The best I could do was call as often as possible until I could get down there. I kept touch with her doctors to make sure things were going the way they should. I also spoke with dad several times a day in hopes to keep his spirits up. My husband was supportive and took care of my 3 young children while I went down to visit. *Doreen*

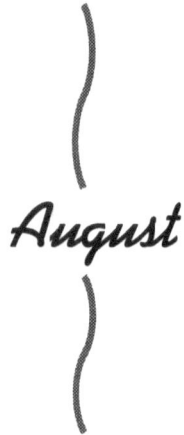

August

August 1, 2003

The start of a new month, boy do the days go by fast. It feels like it was just the start of last month. On the eighth of this month Joan will be getting her third chemo shot and will only have one more to go. We will be very glad when the chemo is all done. I know we have to do the radiation but it will be great to have no more chemo to do. Chemo is the hardest to go through because of all the side effects. Maybe Joan will have some pep after the chemo is done [me too]. Today we did some food shopping. We were starting to run out of things. We have been trying to eat better so we will feel better, they say you are what you eat. Eat junk and you will feel junkie, eat good and you will feel goodie - that doesn't sound right. It must be eat well and you will feel healthy. That's much better. Tonight we had steak, string beans and potatoes for supper. I guess we will feel real healthy by morning – RIGHT! We really are eating better.

PS the days might be going by faster because we sleep half of them.

AUGUST 2 & 3, 2003 - Saturday and Sunday. I'm putting these two days together because both days are just about the same in what we did. Yesterday we got up early because Richard is going to paint the driveway. Richard does anything and everything that you would need to have done around the house - he is a lifesaver for us. He does whatever I can't do any more [just about everything I guess] . Our driveway was OK but was very slippery when it got wet. It needed to have grit put into the paint so we could get some traction when we walked on it. After he finished it on Saturday, the sky opened up and our driveway went down the street and into the sewer. He had to come back today [Sunday] and do it all over again. I know this doesn't have much to do with Joan's problem but it sometimes feels like we went down the sewer drain. Not really - it just feels that way at times. Joan has had some nausea for a few days so it was a good time to do the driveway, we can't drive on it for a few days so we are just staying put until it's all dry. I did leave one car in a parking spot down the street just in case we had to go out. Joan's third chemo shot is due to be done on the eighth of this month only a few days away and I can see the tenseness in Joan's face already. It's not the procedure that worries Joan, it's what happens after. Well enough for today. The early hours we have been getting up for the last two days is catching up to us. talk to you all tomorrow. GOODNIGHT.

August 4, 2003

Today has been a rainy day. It has been raining since yesterday and just does not want to stop. We stayed inside all day. I caught up on more paper work [paper work never seems to stop either] and Joan slept. That chemo really knocks her out. Joan felt OK today, no nausea but still very tired. Joan is eating better which is real good for her. She needs to build up her strength to deal with everything that she is going through. Joan is talking to Rose at this moment which is very good for her mentally. Rose and Joe are very dear to us and we really count on there friendship to get us through this bad time we are going through. We always feel better after talking with them. We hope to see them in late September if Joan is up to the trip to Hilton Head. We would go in between the end of chemo and the start of radiation, and only be there for a few days. I guess we will just have to see how Joan is feeling. Talk to you all tomorrow. Goodnight.

August 5, 2003

Another rainy day, the rainy season is really lasting a long time this year; not only a long time but the amount of rain we are getting is awesome. Most of the time the rainy season consists of about a half hour to an hour every day, and then it would be sunny for the rest of the day. Not this year. It has been raining most all day long for quite awhile. Oh well that's Florida. Joan has been about the same today as she was yesterday, not a lot of nausea but still very tired. Today Joan has stayed in bed most of the day. It could be from the fall she had last night. [Joan has not been to steady on her feet for some time now]. Last night we woke up and had a hard time trying to get back to sleep again. While Joan was getting out of bed, she lost her balance and really went down between the bed and the chair that I was sitting in. I tried to catch her and while I was grabbing her I smacked my head on a picture frame which knocked me backwards into the chair again. Joan was sprawled out on the floor and I on top of the chair. If I had my camera I would have loved to have snapped a picture of us. We could have won some kind of a prize for the most ridiculous pose. We both were stunned and not in too good of shape when we got ourselves up. Joan was aching all over and I had a head that was really hurting. Joan, some how got to the kitchen for the ice pack so I could put it on my head. After an hour we felt a little better and went back to bed. I guess we were just exhausted from our acrobatics that we went right to sleep. We really are OK and will make it through the rest of the night. Talk to you in the morning. Goodnight.

August 6, 2003

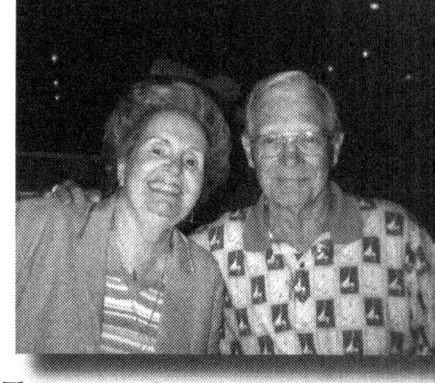

We got up about 10:00 AM and had our breakfast as usual. Joan felt kind of stiff from the fall she had; I was not much better. My head hurt and I also was pretty stiff. Other than that we were not too bad. Joan is not nauseous right now; we will wait to see how the day goes. After hanging out and doing much of nothing, we were feeling a little better. I guess Joan had a bit of pep, so we decided to go to KFC for dinner. There is a real good one close by and we like going there —the food is good and it is very clean. I know Joan has Friday on her mind, and so do I. Neither one of us are looking forward to another chemo session, but we know it is what we must do if Joan is to get all better. Only one more chemo shot after Fridays shot. I'm sure we will be very glad when they are finished. Except for the amount of time the radiation program will take, we feel that we will be in the last inning of Joan being all better. After the radiation is done, maybe we can put things in our life back together again. Let's pray that it goes well and that the time goes quickly.

See you tomorrow.

August 7 & 8, 2003

I put these two days together because Thursday was a nothing day. Really, we did nothing but try to get rid of our aches and pains. Friday we got up early, about 8 AM. Guess we had the chemo appointment on our mind. We had our breakfast and got dressed for the day. Joan put some papers together to bring with us to the Doctor's office. Joan had some questions to ask the Doctor related to her medicines for the nausea. She wanted to know if she should take the nausea pills every day or only when she feels nauseous. The Doctor said she should take the nausea pills about two days before she has the chemo shot and then every day after the shot until the nausea stops. Joan wanted another urine test to see if the urine infection was gone. The results for the urine test was good. The infection was no longer there[Hurray].

I sort of got ahead of myself. The answers to the questions Joan had from the Doctor were after we had gotten to the Doctor's office for the chemo shot. OK, we are now back on track. We arrived at the Doctor's office at 1:30 PM, right on time. We checked in and waited for the nurse to start Joan on the chemo, while we were waiting for the nurse, we had a check up with the Doctor.[At that time Joan had asked her questions and got her answers]. The Doctor said every thing was going OK and we only had one more chemo session after this one, he did not expect any problems and was very positive about everything. He did note that Joan showed positive for being a bit on the anemic side, so he gave Joan a prescription for iron pills to take. After the chemo session, which took about one and a half hours that went pretty fast, because Joan got into conversations with a couple of the other patients. This was very positive for Joan. They were a little ahead of Joan in there programs and were very informative about different things that have happened to them. Again after the chemo session was over we went to dinner on the way home. This was the usual plan because we do not know how Joan will feel starting tomorrow from the chemo. When we got home the sky opened up and the rain really came down hard, so we stayed put and had a quite night.

P.S. Joan was on a high when she was talking to one of the other patients, the other patient took Joan for being 61 or 62 years old and could not believe that Joan was --------------. We will talk to you tomorrow. Goodnight.

August 9, 2003

Joan is now feeling the effects of the chemo a little earlier than the last two times. The last two times Joan did not start feeling any effects of the chemo for a couple of days. This time she started to feel nauseous early this morning [chemo was only done on Friday] Most of today was spent in bed or very close to the bathroom. Joan did not throw up but came close a few times. She also is very flush in the face, but does not have a fever. Her body is aching and she has felt very tired all day. We are not sure whether the aching body is from the fall she had or from the chemo. Joan had a lot of aches in her body from the chemo the last two times. This stage will most likely be with us for most of this week. We were invited to go out to dinner with Rose and Jack tonight, but of course we had to ask for a rain check. Rose and Jack are close friends we have from NJ. They live about ten miles from us here in Florida. We have not seen them for a while for one reason or the other. We will be glad to go to dinner with them when Joan is feeling better. Jack is like a brother to me and always will be. We really enjoy there company. Well it's about time to close this exciting day. We will see you all tomorrow. Goodnight.

August 10, 2003

Today has been a very good day. Nothing to do with our health problems but a lot to do with our family. Kim came home from the Bahamas last night with our three granddaughters. They were there for a week with the Neckle family, most all the women went by plane and all the men went on the Nickel's 28 foot boat. Quite an undertaking especially for the first trip across the ocean. The men including our twelve year old grandson, Justin, came home this morning, safe and sound, THANK GOD. To be very truthful I was not in favor of the boat trip and I am glad it is over and everyone is safe at home. Joan and I had our minds so much on everyone getting home that we almost forgot about Joan not feeling to good. Joan has felt nauseous since the day after her chemo shot and still does today. She has not thrown up at all but feels pretty sick. Of course the wiped out feeling goes along with it also. Joan has been in bed or close to it since Friday and will probably stay that way for the next few days. We have been watching golf for the best part of the day and will most likely stay put in front of the t/v for the rest of the night. Hope Joan starts to feel better to-morrow. Joan has not had much to eat for a few days, but is really not at all hungry for anything. If the stomach does not feel too good it is better you don't put anything into it. Soup, saltines and a bagel are about it for today. Guess I'll close for the day, see you all tomorrow. Goodnight.

August 11, 2003

We are up but not feeling too good. It is about 10:30 AM and Joan is feeling lousy – a lot of nausea and very unsteady on her feet. I made her breakfast, the meal she likes the best, and she could hardly eat it. It is now 4:30 PM and she is eating a grilled cheese and some tapioca pudding or I should say is trying to eat it. Joan has slept most of the day. She is super tired and she is rather flush in the face. She does not have a fever. The temperature in the house is about eighty degrees and Joan is very cold - even to the touch. If you were to touch me you might singe your finger. [only kidding - you'd probably burn it off]. I don't think we will try anything else to eat today, unless she feels like a cup of soup. This time after the chemo shot it seems to be more intense with the nausea and feeling lousy. Oh well, the Doctor said it could be different each time she has the chemo - sure hope it stops soon. Joan is trying very hard to be a good patient and I would say she is doing as well as can be expected. We will probably ride out the rest of the day and then call it quits early. See you tomorrow. Goodnight.

P.S. - Kim was going to come over today, but it is best she waits until another day.

August 12, 2003

Joan seemed to sleep well last night. I for some reason did not. I seemed to be very restless and did not want to keep Joan awake, so I decided to sleep in the guest room. I still had a bad nights sleep - must have had too much on my mind. We both arose about 9:30 AM to start the day. Joan does not feel as nauseous as she did yesterday but she still feels kind of sick to her stomach and is very tired. I know I keep saying that Joan is very tired every day but it is what is happening to her, she just does not have any pep at all and could fall asleep at the snap of a finger. We had breakfast and after lunch I have to go for a chest x-ray at the Martin Memorial Health systems building that is just next door to the Kings Isle Community where we live. I should be back in about one hour. Back from my x-ray. X-ray went well but I sort of took a nose dive before they took the x-ray I sort of lost everything and fell into the bench in a sitting position. Maybe they should be taking a picture of my head instead of my chest. After the x-ray was taken I went home and took the rest of the day off. I still feel a little lightheaded so I will do nothing for the rest of the day. Joan is feeling a little better and is trying to help me - what a team. We will eat something light tonight and maybe go to bed real early. Think I will say goodnight now. If anything of interest happens tonight I will tell you all about it to-morrow. Goodnight.

August 13, 2003

I woke up about 8:00 AM this morning and Joan kept sleeping until about 10:30 AM. Joan seems to be feeling a little better except for her appetite, she still is not eating too well. She just doesn't know what she feels like eating. Nothing seems to be what she would like without feeling nauseous. Yesterday, Joan ate a Taylor ham sandwich for breakfast – nothing for lunch, and a bagel for dinner. She drank a lot of water as she usually does and that was about it. I am sure she will get her appetite back again, but now is when she needs the strength. I will talk to the Doctor about getting her to eat something on a more regular basis. Today is not my day. I feel kind of terrible - my head is killing me. I called the Doctor and she said I should come in at 10:00 AM tomorrow so I will. Today, outside of not eating good Joan seems to be better. We are doing much of nothing today so will see you all tomorrow. Goodnight.

August 14, 2003

Today is an early up day for me, I have to be at the Doctor's office at 10:00 AM to be examined for the hit on the head I got last week. My head is not feeling just right yet and I need to find out what's going on with it. I will not be much help to Joan if I am out of commission. After seeing the Doctor and getting a good exam, the Doctor told me it looked like I have a mild concussion and I need to have a cat scan done on my head. The doctor made an appointment for me to have the cat scan on Friday

the 15th. The doctor told me to go home and take it easy until we find out just what is wrong, if anything. When I got home I told Joan what was said at the Doctor's and we decided that we had better do what the Doctor said. Oh well, life is really full of many exciting things and certainly many surprises. The rest of the day we took it slow and did absolutely nothing. Joan was worried about me, but other than that she felt about the same as yesterday. We have to go to Joan's Doctor for her blood test tomorrow at 1:30 PM . Will let you know how everything works out after we both go to the appointments we have. Have a good night.

August 15, 16 and 17, 2003

Today is the 15th and it is Friday The first appointment was for me for the cat scan. My appointment was at 8:30 AM at the Martin Memorial Building. next to Kings Isle were we live - very convenient. I had the cat scan but will probably hear the results on Monday, another week end wait. Oh well. I'm sure if the results were bad the one who reads it first will get in touch with me right away, or I think that would be what would happen. I went home after the test so I could make breakfast for Joan and myself and then get ready for Joan's blood test at the chemo office. Joan's appointment was at 1:30 PM and we usually like to be there right on time. After they tested Joan's blood they told us that her white count was kind of low and that she was still anemic, which was not good news. Joan has been taking Iron pills for the anemic treatment which was not easy for her to do. The pills upset Joan due to nausea and they had to be taken three times a day - not good. The doctor suggested that Joan take it in a shot form through the port once a week so she would not have to take the pills. This sounded good to both Joan and I. Doing it this way would work well for us, the only draw back was that it will take about one and a half hours to do. What's the difference? We have all kinds of time to spend. I don't think it will effect our social life one bit. We will continue doing it this way until everything is back to normal. We will need to do this once a week on a Friday. Joan felt kind of tired and not too good in the stomach, so we went home. The rest of the day was very quite we just took it easy and thought about what had happened to us on this busy day.

The next day was Saturday the 16th and the only thing we had to do was get ready to go to a birthday party for our granddaughter at Kim's. Our granddaughter would be one year old. We woke up very late this morning, about 11:30 AM. It must have been from being so busy yesterday. Joan did not feel good when she woke up. She was nauseous and every part of her was hurting, OUCH, OUCH, OUCH and OUCH. I on the other hand only had one OUCH but it was a good OUCH. It was my head. The both of us were not in too good of shape. The up side is that we WILL feel good again. When, I'm not too sure, but we know we will get better. Later in the day we had to deal with going to our granddaughter's party, which we both were excited about doing, but not too sure whether we could go with how we felt. It was a hard decision to make but we decided we had better stay home. Neither of us felt good enough to go any place. Joan was nauseous and I had a terrible headache, so we stayed home. SOB, SOB, and double SOB. Kim understood and I'm sure at Siera's age it wasn't a big deal although when she sees us she is always happy we are there. We went to bed early hoping that tomorrow will be a better day.

August 17, 2003

We arose about 10:00 AM. We both felt a little better but Joan not as good as I. Joan still nauseous and very tired and I had, not to bad a headache, but it was still a headache. We again took it easy [I'm tired of saying that]. I went to the store for some fruit. Joan likes fruit more than anything else. This has been a tough session of chemo. I sure hope the fourth and last shot is going to go better than this third one. It has been nine days since the chemo session and Joan does not feel any better. The other two chemo sessions only bothered Joan for about five days. After the five days she felt a little more normal. On the whole, I must say that this experience has been like a bad dream that we know we will wake up from and hope and pray that we won't have the same dream again. I'm tired and I want to go to bed. Goodnight.

August 18 & 19

I am putting these two days together, because I have not really felt like getting on the computer. My eyes and head are still hurting. I am still waiting for my Doctor to call and tell me how the cat scan came out, I guess no news is good news - at least I hope so. Joan has been still feeling nauseous and aching all over, she has eaten a little better in the last two days, than she has in a long time. That is really a good sign and I hope she continues. Even though she is still feeling nauseous she seems to want something to eat. Maybe being hungry is taken over the feeling of nausea. Maybe it is the not eating that is also making Joan nauseous. ???? I hate to say it but we just took it easy for the rest of the two days. I will continue our episode tomorrow. Goodnight.

August 20, 2003

Joan and I awoke about 9:30 AM this morning, had breakfast and got dressed for the day. The only thing on our agenda for today is Joan's appointment with Sheila, Joan's nail person.. Joan would not miss this appointment for anything. After we had Joan's nails done we went next door to the Jewelers to get a pair of earrings for Sierra, who was one year old on the 10th of August. Sierra has to get her ears pierced, so she can wear the earrings. Kim will have that done soon. Joan is still not feeling well, but is better than she was yesterday. We finally got out of the house and did something besides REST. Maybe we will go out again tomorrow. Doreen, our lovely daughter, is coming to see us for about five days and we are very excited about having her here. We need to get a few things from the store so it will be our chance to get out again. There is nothing going on with the Doctor's for Joan until Friday, when she goes for her blood check and to get her iron shot for the week. I'll let you know how we do. Talk to you tomorrow. Goodnight.

August 21, 2003

Today is the day before Doreen gets here, and we are very excited knowing that she will be here. Joan feels so-so, not to good, but not to bad. I think she is starting to feel a little better, like before her last shot. I sure hope so as she certainly has had a rough time the last two weeks. We are hoping that her last shot in September will be a lot easier. I guess what ever happens will happen and we will cope with it as we always do. I guess I should have waited until the night was finished. Joan just took her temperature and it was a shade under 101 degrees. That is not a high temperature but with her immune system not being too good, it worries us. Joan took a couple of Motrin to reduce the fever, and about two hours later her temperature was back to normal, thank God. A fever is not what you want when you are on chemo. We will take it again when we wake up in the middle of the night, which we always do. We will tell you what it was tomorrow. Goodnight.

August 22, 2003

Joan's temperature was normal when we woke up in the middle of last night. I guess the temperature Joan had was not a serious problem, thank God. Today Joan is due to go to the Doctor's office in Stuart, for her iron shot which she gets every Friday. While we were there the Doctor decided to check out Joan having a temperature. Well, I guess that was a good idea, because Joan's immune system was way below what it should be. Her system could no longer fight off any infections that she might get. The Doctor ordered medicine to give Joan, to build up her white cell count. This took about one half hour to do along with the time for her iron shot. I guess her fever the other night was more serious then we thought. You really never know how bad something could be so it was a good thing to run things past the Doctor when we saw him. Don't take chances, check everything out whether you think it's a problem or not. Joan must be very careful with every thing she does from now on - meaning do not go near any one who even looks like they are sick. Keep washing your hands and do not touch anything that has even a remote chance of having germs on it. The medicine should clear up the problem, but it might take a while to do so. For as long as Joan is on chemo this could be a real bad problem so we are going to be super careful with every thing that we do. This is not something to fool with. When we got home we had to get ready for our daughter Doreen's arrival. Thank God she was getting here today as we really needed something to cheer us up and she sure can

do that. Doreen arrived safe and sound and we are now going to just sit back and enjoy her being with us. We will talk again tomorrow. We are very busy enjoying our daughter. Goodnight.

August 23 & 24, 2003

Saturday and Sunday were both about the same as far as Joan's condition. She felt pretty good except for being tired, and having a little bit of a headache. I had a problem with my left leg, which swelled up and was a bit uncomfortable. Doreen took care of both problems, she put Mom in the closet after giving her two sleeping pills. She also took care of me. She put ice on my leg and also gave me two sleeping pills. The only thing she forgot to do was to take the ice out of the refrigerator after putting it on my leg. BBBBRRRRrrrrrrrrrrr. We had two good days with our daughter Doreen. She is so nice to have around, especially if you don't feel good. She just knows what to do. We are going to watch a video on the t/v so will talk to you tomorrow.

Goodnight.

August 25, 2003

We all awoke a little late - must have stayed up too late last night. Joan felt pretty good, just tired as she usually is due to the chemo. Doreen and I felt OK but also were tired but not due to chemo. Joan seems to be getting over her nausea feeling and is feeling a bit better. The nauseous feeling lasted a good three and one half weeks since her last shot. That's about twice as long as it has ever lasted. Hopefully the next and last chemo procedure will not be as bad. Joan's aches and pains have not been as bad as they were. Hopefully this is a turn for the better. We have been having a good time being with our daughter Doreen but we feel real bad that our daughter Kim has not been able to be with us due to her not feeling well. We were afraid that with Joan's immune system so low that it was not a good idea for Joan to be near any one with a cold. We know Kim agrees and that she understands for her Mom's sake. All our children have been very supportive and would do anything to make their Mom better. We love all our children and know the feeling is mutual. We are a close family and when one of us is sick or has a problem we all feel it and will do anything to help. Tomorrow is Doreen's last day visiting us so we are going to pack every minute with being with her. I'll say goodnight now. Goodnight.

August 26, 2003

Doreen's last day before going back to NJ. We all got up about 8:30 AM to start the day. After breakfast we sat around and talked and went over all the things that our daughter Doreen thought we should do, she has excellent ideas and we will try to mend some of our ways to include some of the things she thought we should be doing. All of our children give us good advice and we try to incorporate what they suggest into our daily living. This is how our family stays so close. We are not afraid to communicate with one another. We are always very comfortable with giving all our children advice even at their age, they will always listen to what we say and try to fit our suggestions into their ways. After talking for a while we decided to go to Rotties for lunch. Rotties is a restaurant on Hutchinson Island right on the ocean, it overlooks the beach and ocean and is a very lovely place to go - the view is just wonderful. Joan insisted that Doreen and I go. Doreen has never been there. We did go and we had a wonderful time.

Doreen just loved Rotties and said she would make it a definite stop for her and her family to go when she is here again. When we got home

Joan had just woke up from a nap that she usually takes in the afternoon. We hung around the house and relaxed until suppertime. About 7:30 PM Doreen met Kim at Friendlys for ice cream and a short visit. Kim has not been coming to our house while she has the cold, it made all of us unhappy but was a necessary precaution for Joan's condition. I have been talking a lot about things that we have been doing that are not about Joan's condition but really they are connected. It is all part of our family's concern about Joan and is our family's way of being together when there is a problem. We are going to bed early because Doreen is being picked up by the limo to take her to the airport at 7:30 a.m. Will talk to you all tomorrow.

Goodnight.

August 27, 2003

Another early morning - up at 6:00 AM this morning. We had to rise early because our daughter, Doreen was leaving for home today. We know she needs to get home to her husband and children, and we know that's the way it has to be, but there should be a law that when your children get married they have to spend at least every other month with there parents. I think I have lost it or maybe I'm just getting senile. Really, we had a wonderful five days with Doreen. We didn't do anything but hang around the house and have Doreen visit with her Mom. Joan really needed Doreen to be here to pick up her spirits. That is just what Doreen did. She also was a great help to both Joan and myself. It was so special because it was undivided attention that Doreen was able to give. We adore our grandchildren but it isn't very often when you can have a daughter all to your self for any length of time. All our children are very, very busy with all our grandchildren as it should be. But I'll say it again, IT WAS REAL SPECIAL. We would like to do it with all our children. [Don't push it Dad.] After Doreen left we just hung around thinking about the nice time we had. Joan is feeling pretty good today, no nausea, just tired. This Friday Joan has To go to the Doctor's for a blood test. It seems like we just did that. Joan has to be checked regularly for the white cell count which has been to low and has affected Joan's immune system. We also have to go for the chemo shot next week on the fourth of September. Here we go again. Doreen arrived home at her home in Ramsey, NJ safely and with out any trouble. The only thing was the amount of time it took to do so, Doreen left our house at 7:30 AM and arrived at her house in Ramsey NJ at 6:00 PM. That's just a shade under twelve hours for what should be a three hour flight from Florida to New Jersey. The nine extra hours were spent getting to the airports and the waiting time at each airport for security and boarding time. The time it took was long but we could not be any happier because she arrived at her home safely. Our many prayers were answered. I guess it is time for us to go to bed so I will talk to you all tomorrow. Goodnight.

August 28, 2003

Today was real weird. I woke up about 6:00 AM but had no idea why so I decided to try and go back to sleep. It worked and believe it or not I did not wake up again until 11:30 AM. I could not believe my eyes when I looked at the clock. What's even more bazaar was that Joan woke up the same time 11:30 AM without first waking up at 6:00 AM. The whole morning was over and we were both still tired. All I can say is we must really have needed the sleep. Joan felt OK but decided to spend the rest of the day just hanging out in the bed. I had to get a hair cut at 1:30 PM, so that meant I had to get moving. I get my hair cut at the same place Joan gets her hair done. Everyone at the salon was glad to see me and wanted to hear all about how Joan was doing

All at the salon are real beautiful people and we mean that from the bottom of our hearts. They treat us like real friends not just customers. We love all of them very much. Neil, who is the owner, is very good to Joan. He always wants to know weather he can do anything for Joan and he sends her flowers, like every month, from all at the salon. I'm going to fertilize Joan's head to help the growing process of Joan's hair just so she can go there real soon. After my hair cut we spent the rest of the day - Joan sleeping and watching t/v and me doing some paper work and reading. We had supper and just went back to what we were doing before. It is now time for bed so I'll say Goodnight. Goodnight. P.S. We sure miss our daughter being here.

August 29, 2003

Today we got up at 9:30 AM, took an early shower and ate breakfast. We did all of this before we had to leave for Joan's appointment with Doctor Iannotti for her blood test and her iron shot, which was at 2:45 PM. [Are we speedy or what?] This was an important appointment. We would be finding out about Joan's immune system, her white blood cell count and her iron count. No. 1, Joan's immune system, which was very low at .07, needed to be a lot higher or she would be in big trouble. We were very excited because it went to 2.09. This does not mean she is out of the woods yet, but it is a big step in the right direction. Joan must still keep away from any one or any thing that could give her any kind of sickness or infections. No. 2, Joan's white blood cell count was improved and also her iron level was a bit better. Joan has the final chemo session on the fourth of September next Tuesday, so we really have to be careful, the chemo really can do a job on the immune system. The Doctor and nurses have done a great job on correcting any problems that have come up since Joan has been on the chemo program. Our faith in God is really what has been keeping us going. Also all the prayers and support from our family and our real close friends who are just like family. We also have prayers coming from people that we do not even know and have heard about Joan being sick. We thank everyone who has taken the time and thoughtfulness to care about what happens to us. We love you and pray for you all. In this world of ours, knowing what is going on, it sure is a wonderful feeling to have so many human beings that care for one another. This is a good world that we were given. It just needs us all to get back on track and start living the kind of life that was intended for us to live. On our way home from the Doctor's, we stopped at the Red Lobster Restaurant for dinner. We thought it would be OK because it was about four PM and there were not many people inside yet. We had a good dinner, and being out was just what we needed. We ordered a bunch of crab legs, steak and salad. What a ball we had. I think we needed a shower when we got home, it sure was messy but OH SO GOOD. After dinner we went home and relaxed until bed time. It was a good day. Goodnight.

August 30 and 31, 2003

Might as well put in September 1, 2003 for the whole Labor Day Weekend. Well, I guess we started the week end by getting up at our pretty normal time on Saturday, the 30th, which is between 9:00 AM and 10:00 AM. We had breakfast and got ourselves ready to start the Labor Day weekend. Normally, if Joan were OK, we would most likely have been in PA at our son's house or in NJ at our daughter Doreen's house, looking forward to at least three cook outs; one at our son's house, one at our daughter Doreen's house and one at our daughter Diane's house. We would have enjoyed all the cook outs and being with all our children in the North. When you are dealt the cards you must play out the hand you were dealt, and that is what we are doing. We are very fortunate that we have our Daughter Kim and her whole family by our side, even though we can not visit very much because of Joan's problem with her immune system being so low. We can't take the chance of Joan getting sick from anyone that might be sick. We are very lucky that we can be by ourselves alone and get along so well, I guess it is something that we were always able to do, even when we were not sick. Maybe that is the secret of being married for FIFTY YEARS. We do miss being with others, but we know that as soon as this period is over and Joan is OK things will get back to normal.

Sunday and Monday were pretty much the same as Saturday, taking it easy and watching a lot of t/v especially the golf which was on all three days. Joan does not play golf but she enjoys watching it on the t/v. [Yeah Tiger] We talked to a lot of family and friends on the phone the whole weekend, which was real good for both of us. We are not forgotten just lost for a short time. Only kidding - we know exactly where we are, just don't know how we got here. Joan is not as nauseous as she has been but is very tired as she has been. I guess the being tired is going to last as long as she is on the chemo program. We understand that the radiation will make her tired also. I think we will close now, but will be up and at em first thing in the morning [ya right]. Goodnight

Voice of the Children

How did you deal with your own fears?

Of course I asked the question - could this happen to me? All I can do is take all the precautions available and pray. I only hope that this will not strike anyone else in our family after seeing what my parents had to go through. *Diane*

I tend to keep my fears and emotions bottled up inside. I know I had fears but I'm not sure how to put into words how it affected me. *Ken*

September

September 2, 2003

The holiday is over, and it's hard to believe that it is September already. It seems like the summer has just not existed, maybe because we simply haven't paid too much attention to it. We started with Joan's problem in March and it has been like a never ending merry go round that just does not want to stop. Joan has one more chemo session which is this Thursday at 1:30 PM. I'm sure there will be a lot of things we will be told by Doctor Iannotti and his staff. Joan will most likely have to keep coming back to the cancer center until she no longer has to have the iron shots and until her immune system is back on track. Once Joan is released from Doctor Iannotti's care, which probably won't be until late September or the beginning of October, she will most likely start with the radiation program. The radiation treatments are on the first floor of the same building that we have been coming to for the chemo. This is all part of the cancer center in Stuart FL. Joan will be taking radiation treatments everyday except Saturday and Sunday for about six weeks, or so we've been told. Anything can be changed at any time as we well know, so it is better to just wait and see what takes place - when it takes place. [Hope that sounded right, if not, oh well.] Other than what I said, so far the day has been a restful one. The only thing we did today that was different was to get Joan's nails done. I think Joan would have to be in the desert with no way to travel to miss her nail appointment. She did not feel just right while at the nail solon so it was right home to lie down after she was finished. We will have supper, watch t/v and go to bed so I will be back at you tomorrow. Goodnight.

September 3, 2003

Up at 10:00 AM, showered, dressed and had breakfast. We took today to go over all our thoughts of what has happened, and what is going to happen as far as Joan's situation about her illness. Thursday is Joan's last chemo session, which in our minds brings up a lot of questions we must ask the Doctor. We know it will be a while before we start the radiation sessions. Joan has to get over all the symptoms of the chemo treatment, before we start with the radiation - at least that is what we were led to believe. Joan and I know she could not handle the two treatments at the same time. We believe they will not start anything else until Joan feels better from all the chemo in her system, and her blood levels are where they should be. And, of course, her immune system should be all corrected. I guess we should just wait and not try to second guess the program. I'm sure the Doctor will do what is right. I guess it is only natural for us to be a little apprehensive about what is in store for us. We know what's coming but do not know when it is to happen. I'm sure at some point they will do something to find out if the cancer is truly gone and I'm sure that is deep down what both of us are thinking about. I know we truly believe that the cancer is gone and that the Doctor's are also sure but I guess we just have to have some kind of proof that it is. We will go through the rest of today thinking about all these things and come up with just what we want to know from the Doctor tomorrow. Tussling with our thought is becoming old hat to us, and it is good that we communicate with one another about what we are individually thinking. It helps us to discuss it rather than keep it all inside until an explosion takes place. I think we will sign off now and let you now how everything comes out tomorrow. Goodnight.

September 4, 2003

It is now "tomorrow" and we are getting ourselves ready to go to see the Doctor. Yes, we got up, took a shower, and ate breakfast first. Today is also the day that Carol comes to clean. She was a little late getting here but that is not a problem because she can lock up after we leave. We need to leave at 1:00 PM to be at the Doctor's office by 1:45 PM. It was a real long session today, seeing that it was the fourth and last chemo session. We will still have to go to Doctor Iannotti for blood tests and Iron shots, also he will still be keeping track of Joan for quite a while. Joan's immune system will still need to be watched until it is where it should be. Also, Joan will need the iron shots until she is no longer anemic. For the next two weeks we will have to go to see the Doctor to see how Joan is doing. Then it will be ounce a month check ups for at least three months. When Joan is pretty much back to normal the check ups will be twice a year until whenever. This is a good thing. I asked Doctor Iannotti if the cancer was all gone thinking I would get a yes or no answer. Instead he said the cancer that Joan had from the tumor is gone but that Joan will have to be very aware of what is going on in her body. Once you've had cancer you seem to be at a high risk of getting it again, so you need to be very careful. Joan will get a call from Doctor Griffis office to set up an appointment for the start of radiation. We are now at home after a long day at the Doctor's. We are very tired and cannot wait to go to bed. Joan feels not too bad right now, but she can feel the Nausea starting to kick in. [Here we go.] We hope we will have a better month than the one we just finished. I'll say goodnight now and be with you tomorrow when I can make more sense out of what happened today. Goodnight.

September 5, 2003

This is the day after Joan's last chemo session. We slept kind of OK last night, but we did have some restless moments. We talked for a little while and than went back to sleep. Joan does not feel to well today. She is very nauseous and just feels sick. I guess it is going to be like last month. Oh well, we got through last month somehow, so I guess we can do it again. Joan is kind of flush in the face but does not have a fever. We take Joan's temperature at least twice a day to be on the safe side. Joan has not been able to eat very much today, her food intake was a couple of bites out of her Taylor ham sandwich, which is her favorite meal. Lunch consisted of two saltine crackers and supper was half a bowl of chicken noodle soup. That was it for the day. [She did keep everything down but just barely.] Joan does drink a lot of water, like eight, eight ounce glasses every day. I'm sure that keeps her from getting dehydrated which is important. In talking to Doctor Iannotti, the chemo Doctor, we now have a good idea on just what is going to take place in the coming months and it also gives us an idea on just how long Joan will be in treatment.. It looks as if no cancer shows up in the next five years we can be almost sure that she will not have any more trouble concerning cancer. We will always have to be on the look out for anything that might show up though. We are both still pretty tired so

I'm sure we will turn in early tonight. I had a Doctor appointment today with the dermatologist for a couple of pre-cancer spots on my body, nothing serious just a routine check up. I went when Joan was sleeping and I was back in about one hour. I do not like leaving Joan alone but Kim will keep a check on her while I am gone. We are still very positive that everything is going to turn out OK. With all our prayers and every one else's prayers, how can we miss? Some times you might wonder if God hears your prayers, but believe me he hears all the prayers and he does take care of every one of them. It is getting late so I think I'll end the day and go to bed. Joan has already done so. Goodnight.

September 6, 2003

Today is not much different from yesterday, Joan feels about the same. We woke up about 8:30 AM but laid in bed until almost 10:00 AM, I made Joan her Taylor ham sandwich for breakfast and to my surprise she ate the whole thing, and said it was very good. We did not do much for the rest of the day except talk and watch t/v. I can always find paperwork to do so that's just what I did for about an hour. Joan was taking a nap or at least it looked like she was. About 4:00 PM I made Joan a dish of macaroni and cheese for what we call a late lunch or an early supper. Joan ate it all up, again much to my surprise, and she seemed to enjoy it. About an hour later Joan started to get real nauseous and that is how she stayed until near midnight when she through up. Joan does not throw up to often but stays on the verge of doing so constantly. After Joan threw up she seemed to feel a lot better but was real tired and totally wiped out to the point of not being able to walk without my help or she would just fall down. Well that takes care of today so its off to bed we go. Goodnight.

September 7, 2003

We woke up about 9:00 AM and just laid in bed until almost 10:30 AM waiting to see how Joan was going to feel. Joan felt a little better or so it seemed so we got out of bed and had our breakfast. Joan still felt a little better but began to feel that old feeling of nausea coming back. It looks like it will be another day just like yesterday. We hope not. We will just see how it goes. It is now about 3:30 PM and Joan now has a good case of nausea. We kind of slid past lunch and thought it better to just have some supper and call it quits as far as eating goes. Supper consisted of a good bowl of vegetable soup [the old fashion kind with just vegetables]. It seemed to be the right choice and tasted pretty good to both of us. Joan still has the nausea but was able to keep everything down. We did not want to press our luck, so we just hung out in the bedroom until it was time to go to bed. Hope tomorrow will find Joan feeling better. That's all for today folks. Goodnight.

September 8, 2003

Today we got out of bed at 10:00 AM, had breakfast and got ready for what ever this new day brings us. Hopefully it will be a day that Joan will not be nauseous, at least not as much as she has been. We also hope that it will be the start of Joan starting to get better from all the side effects that the chemo has given her. It is a day that I have to go to my heart Doctor for a check up, and to ask him some important questions about what is coming up for me medically. I must take good care of my self so I can be of help to Joan. I will most likely need an operation for a hernia on the left side in the groin area. It is something that has bothered me for a month or two and the Doctor said if I am careful I could do it when Joan gets better. That sounds good to me, because I am not going to do anything at all but take care of my wife until she is all better. She must be all done with her chemo and its side effects, her radiation and any side effects it might have, before I will venture into anything for me short of a real emergency. I know I get tired and sometimes a little short of energy but that is what Joan and I have always been about. We take care of each other and it is not all one sided. I have had my problems and Joan has had to be the care taker for me. We do it not as a job or something that we are expected to do, we do it because we just can't stand to see one or the other suffer. It must be that we have been together so long that when one of us hurts it hurts the other - and neither of us likes hurting. I had a good report from my check up today. The Doctor said everything looks OK and that my heart could stand a minor operation, like the hernia operation, if it had to be done. That is very good news. I got home from the Doctor's about 3;30 PM and Joan and I just hung out and talked about what the Doctor told me. We had supper around 6;00 PM and settled in for the night. We will again go to bed early - for us that is about 12:00 PM. Will talk to you tomorrow. Goodnight.

September 9, 2003

Today we should hear from Doctor Griffis's office about an appointment for Joan to start her radiation. The call came late morning, and we set an appointment for next Monday, the 15th at 12:30 PM. This appointment will not be for the beginning of the radiation, but will be to talk to the Doctor and get all of the preliminaries out of the way, such as drawing the road map on Joan showing where the radiation will be going. We don't know exactly how they do it, but AM sure they do. The radiation will most likely start in about two weeks, after Joan has recovered from her chemo program. That will bring us near the end of September to start the radiation and would go right through October and into the first week of November. We will see what we will see. Today other than make the appointment we just discussed everything and hung out. Our Daughter Kim stopped in to visit with our Granddaughter, Sierra, who we haven't seen up close in about four weeks. We cant tell you how much we really enjoyed being with the both of them. We did not do hugs and kisses to be on the safe side, but we thoroughly enjoyed the visit. We did have lunch. Joan does not feel too bad today but had that nausea feeling all the time. After Kim and Sierra left, which was about 2:15 PM, we just rested and I think we both fell asleep for a short time. After our little siesta we thought about supper and what to have. I guess I push a little about Joan eating. It sort of upsets Joan and I get real, frustrated. I think we both counted to ten about ten times and decided not to discuss it at all. I had something to eat and I'll bet Joan will wait until it is ice cream time and forget all about dinner. I got that right, oh well, at least she will get some dairy products in the ice cream. Joan needs to have a better diet than she has if she wants to get her strength back. WE WILL WORK ON THAT - NOT TONIGHT, BUT WE WILL WORK ON IT. We had a big hug and kiss and both went to bed. Goodnight.

September 10, 2003

Today looks like one of those nothing days. I can not think of anything that we are to do, probably because we have nothing to do. Joan feels kind of nauseous but not real sickish, of course she is very tired and feels very weak in the legs. I have a couple of projects to do so that will fill up part of the day for me. Joan has no projects to do except to keep track of me, which she does because she is always worried that I am going to do something that would not be good for me health-wise. I can't knock that because it is out of love for me that she does it. After I finished my projects we watched a little news on the t/v, there is a new hurricane brewing out in the Atlantic and we always like to see just where it is going. Hopefully it is going to stay out in the Atlantic. We will pray that it does - join us please.

Today we had three pretty good meals, no discussions before. I just made them. For breakfast Joan had her usual Taylor ham on roll with orange juice. I had my cereal. For lunch, Joan had a grilled cheese sandwich and a Coke. I had a tuna sandwich and a glass of milk. For supper, we both had a loin of pork with string beans and a baked potato. Pretty good, I'd say. I think we will just take one day at a time and see how we do. We will not plan meals - just make them and see what happens. The rest of the day we just did our usual - t/v and go to bed. See you tomorrow. Goodnight.

September 11, 2003

Today we have an appointment with Doctor Iannotti to have a blood test, an iron shot and to check out Joan's immune system. We were about ready to go and Joan said that she did not feel good at all. Joan felt real nauseous and just about ready to throw up. I decided to call the Doctor's office and try to cancel today's appointment and re-schedule one for tomorrow. I talked to the nurse and she said it would be no problem to do so. Joan now has an appointment at 1:45 PM on tomorrow. It is real important that Joan has this all done every week and sometimes twice in one week if she is not feeling well. Now that we straightened that all out, I'll tell you about the rest of the day. Yep, you got it, we just hung around and waited to see if Joan was going to throw up. While we waited Joan slept, or I should say she tried to sleep, and I just waited with her. I really could not start much of anything the way Joan felt, so I got plenty of rest just doing nothing. We will eat dinner and do our normal night time activities. Do I have to say it? Oh, OK - we watched t/v and went to bed. Goodnight.

September 12, 2003

After I said goodnight last night, Joan got real sick, she threw up and really felt like she went through a ringer. This all happened about 11:00 PM just a little after going to bed. When Joan was all cleaned up, we went back to bed and fell asleep. Joan was really wiped out and to tell you the truth, so was I. It was a hard day.

Today we got up about 7:30 AM. Joan seemed to feel a little better but not to sure just how much. Joan decided to stay in bed for awhile, I guess she really does not feel that great. I had a cup of coffee and went out side to put on the water for my gardens, seeing that it hasn't really rained that much in the past few days. We need to get ready to go to the Doctor this afternoon at 1:45 PM. This is in place of the appointment we missed yesterday. It is very important that we make this appointment so we will give it a real effort to do so. As we were getting dressed to go to the Doctor Joan said that she didn't think she could make it. She felt just like she was going to throw up. We sat down and tried to figure out just what might happen if we did not go. After thinking about it and knowing that it was Friday and all of the Doctor's would not be in until Monday, we decided that we had better really try and go. We packed up a bag with the items Joan would need if she were to get sick on the way, things like a bucket, a towel, and a change of clothes and a bottle of water. After packing all of these things we got in the car and off to the Doctor's we went. On the way Joan just looked worse and I could not wait until we got there. We arrived at the Doctor's in about forty five minutes. That's about how long it usually takes to get there. When I got Joan out of the car, she could not stand on her feet. She was very weak and getting worse every second. I sat Joan down in the car and went to get a wheel chair. I put Joan in the wheel chair and off we went again. I got her to the Doctor's office and the nurse took over rather quickly. Doctor Iannotti looked at Joan right away and told the nurse to start the I.V. going right away. They gave Joan seven different things through the I.V. - all of which she needed very badly. No 1 - Intravenous feeding; No 2 - Iron; No 3 - Sedative; No 4 - Medicine to increase her white blood cells which were very, very low; No 5 - Medicine for her immune system which was also very low; No 6 -Medicine to help her with the nausea; and No 7 - A saline solution to clean out the Port. This all took about two to two and a half hours to do. I do not know what we would of done if we had decided not to go to the Doctor's. All I can say is God was with us all the way with the decision that we made.

Joan really fell apart when we got into the Doctor's office, she started to cry and really needed to be calmed down or she would have hyperventilated - so the Doctor said. After Joan felt better we left for home - and I mean straight home. Neither of us could wait to get there. After arriving home we thanked God for turning a bad situation into a good outcome.

Joan was like a different person from the person that I took to the Doctor. I think we will just take it easy the whole weekend until we go back to the Doctor's office on Monday. The Doctor we are seeing on Monday will be Doctor Griffis, the radiologist. He is in the same building as Doctor Iannotti. They all work together but on different floors. I think it is time for us to just say goodnight and go to bed. Goodnight.

September 13, 2003

Got up early this morning. Don't know why we just did. It was 6:30 AM. I stayed up and Joan went back to sleep until 9:00 AM - still don't have a clue why so early. We had nothing scheduled for today except Luise was going to come about noon time to prepare the house for the hurricane that might come our way. We sure hope it does not hit Florida or any other state anywhere. It is a very powerful storm and would do much damage. So far it looks like it will miss us and there is a good chance it might go out to sea. I really hope so. Maybe if we all prayed to God that it will make that turn to the Northeast it just might happen. Let's at least give it a shot - I know I will. Today, Joan, outside of being real tired, is feeling much better than she was yesterday. She is like a different person, and is even doing things around the house - not much but it's a start. She was working on the photo albums, putting them in order and she did a pretty good job of it. She has started to eat a little better, and that really makes me very happy. She really needs to be a lot stronger than she is, and that will come I'm sure from eating right. Today and tomorrow will be kind of a get it together time. We have to go to the Doctor's Monday and it would be nice if Joan could show them at the Doctor's office how much better she is doing. I was scared Friday. I thought Joan was going to have a seizure or a heart attack. It really reminded me of when she was in the hospital last year and had a seizure. So much for that. Joan is going to be OK from now on and the other day is going to stay in the past. PERIOD. Well guys, I think I will head for the bedroom and call it a night. We had a pretty good day considering. Goodnight.

September 14, 2003

Today is just what I thought it would be - rest, rest, and more rest. We did not get up until 11:30 AM. Could be because we had a restless night and didn't get a whole lot of sleep. This happens to us quite often, it might be because we are not too active and the body is not tired enough. The mind is saying lets go to sleep but the body is saying not now. Joan feels better as far as the nausea goes, but is having trouble with her tongue. It is called Rush and is one of the side effects from the chemo. It is a little raw and hurts when she swallows. This is just what we need. Joan hasn't noticed it too much when she was so nauseous but it is bothering her now. Whatever side effects comes with taking chemo, Joan was almost sure to get them. Joan has medicine to take for the Rush on her tongue, but I think the chemo was not letting it do what it was supposed to do. Joan had her fourth and last chemo shot so maybe now the medicine for the Rush will start to do what it is supposed to do. I sure hope so.

The rest of today will most likely be spent doing a lot of nothing but watching t/v and taking cat naps. Oh yes, we still have to figure out dinner. What do we do about dinner. I thought it was hard to come up with a suggestion for what Joan would like to eat before the Rush became a problem. Now it is going to be next to impossible to figure out. Maybe she could go on an ice cream diet. That would go down with not too much of a problem and look at all the choices she would have with all the flavors they make, and all the different ways to make it. Oh well, I'm sure we will figure it all out and Joan will not starve. I think I will say goodnight for today but will talk to you tomorrow.

Goodnight.

September 15, 2003

Joan is still not feeling up to par and seems pretty, as she calls it, wobbly. She just does not have any strength, I talked to Doctor Iannotti on the phone today and he said that Joan was having a hard time with all that is going on with her. He believes that the medicines she got last Friday should be kicking in by now. These medicines are to increase her white blood cell count and to build her immune system up, also to increase her iron so she will not be anemic and would give her the strength she needs. Doctor Iannotti said if she does not improve soon I am to call him again and he would consider blood transfusions for Joan. We hope it does not come to that, but will do what ever it takes to get Joan better. I don't think what is going on with Joan is the norm. I think it is because she has gotten almost all the side effects from the chemo. Aren't we lucky. We will get through this with God's help, I am sure. We will finish out the rest of today and get back to you all tomorrow. OK? Goodnight.

September 16, 2003

Today we got up about 9:30 AM, showered, had breakfast and started the day. Nothing really on today's schedule so we thought we would just hang out and see how Joan would feel as the day went on. Yesterday, Doctor Iannotti told me that the medicines Joan got on Friday of last week should be kicking in by now and that she will start to feel better. I guess we will just wait and see if it does. It is now mid-afternoon and by crackey Joan does seem better. I guess the Doctor knows what he is doing. The rest of the day we just had dinner and talked to our kids up North. They were a little concerned about hurricane Isabel and to where it was going. Joan still feels OK and we are hoping she will continue to feel better until she is ALL better. Time to say goodnight. Goodnight.

September 17, 2003

GOOD NEWS! Joan woke up and feels pretty good. What a nice way to start the day. Today we have a couple of things on the schedule. Joan has a nail appointment and I have an appointment with the eye Doctor for a check up. Joan's appointment is at 1:00 PM and mine is at 1:45 PM. They are only two minutes away from each other so I will be able to go to my appointment while Joan is having hers. We did not finish with our appointments until after 3:30 PM and then went right home. Joan still feeling OK. We received a call from Doctor Griffis at about 4:30 PM to confirm Joan's appointment tomorrow and to tell us to go to Doctor Iannotti's office first for a blood test. I guess he wants to be sure that Joan's blood levels are OK. The rest of the day was spent just enjoying Joan feeling better. Anything that is a plus for Joan puts us on cloud nine or so it seems. We had a good dinner and retired early. That means we went to bed and watched t/v until we fell asleep. Goodnight.

September 18, 2003

It's still a good morning. Joan is feeling OK and that of course is what is making it a good morning. We have had breakfast and have gotten dressed for the day. We waited for Carol, the cleaning lady, to come and then we got ready to go to the Doctor's. After Carol left, we left for the Doctor's office to have Joan's blood taken and checked. We left about 1:00 PM and arrived at Doctor Iannotti's office at 2:00 PM. It took us a little longer than usual; why, I don't really know - must have been the traffic. The nurse took Joan's blood and had the report made up and given to us by 2: 20 PM. They knew we had an appointment with Doctor Griffis at 2:30 PM, so they got on it right away. The report was very good as far as the white blood cell count goes. It came out normal which meant that Joan's immune system was right on target. It is the first time since Joan was on the chemo treatment. The reading for the red blood cell count was not so good. It was lower than it was at the last reading. The red blood cells - being low meant that the iron count was too low and Joan was still anemic which is not too good. If the iron does not correct itself by Friday, the Doctor said we would have to consider having a blood transfusion. I sure hope that we won't have to do that. We went down to the first floor for our appointment with Doctor Griffis. We were going to have a roadmap put on Joan's body. Seriously, they have to mark all the spots where she has to have radiation done. It is quite a complicated procedure that is done with a computer and marked like she was having a tattoo in all the spots for the radiation treatment. This complete procedure takes about two hours to do, but wouldn't you know, the computer broke and Joan had to get out of the machine until they fixed it. After it was fixed, Joan went back into the machine and they finished the procedure. That delay took about an extra hour to the length of the procedure. [The machine, as I call it looks just like a cat scan, and I really do not know just what they call it. I'll find out and let you know later].

With the delay, we now are at 5:30 PM and we are very tired and want to go home. We went over everything with the nurse and made some more appointments for next week. I do not think they will start the radiation treatments for at least two to three weeks from now, at least we don't think so. I guess we will really know after Joan's next blood test on the 26th of this month. It took us about an hour to get home and we still had to have dinner. We put some left-over pizza in the oven and called that dinner. We than went to bed and - you know what - watched t/v until we fell asleep. See you all tomorrow. Goodnight. [I'm too tired to go on.]

September 19, 2003

We had a very restless time last night. We must have gotten up at least three times. I guess we were overtired from the busy day we had. We did not get up this morning until 11:30 AM. I guess we should have lunch instead of breakfast. Sounds good to me. After we ate, we talked about what we did yesterday at the Doctor's office and tried to understand exactly what we are doing. After looking at the papers, I think we have a handle on every thing. It always seems to be too much to handle, but somehow we do get the strength to do it. I think we know where our strength really comes from. He never fails us. We do not have anything on the schedule this week until next Friday. I guess it gives us a lot of time to get ready for what ever will come next. I think we are getting worn out and getting the feeling that all these things will never end. With a few days off and nothing to do we should feel better and be all set to go again. Joan feels pretty good today but seems to have a lot of aches and pains from the workout she received at the Doctor's office - going through the procedure, to get ready for radiation. They really did draw a road map on her body. We did very little for the rest of the day, I had some paper work to do and Joan just rested. We will eat dinner and I AM positive we will turn in early, so I'll say goodnight now. Goodnight.

How We Feel Up to Now

From the day we were told that Joan had cancer of the breast, 3/31/03, I would have to say that we are still in a state of not believing what we were told, and what we have gone through for the last seven months. The time has really gone very fast, thank God. It seems like just yesterday that we were told the bad news. Our lives have really changed. Not that we were so active before, from doing what we wanted to do, when we wanted to do it, to being told what to do when ever we were told to do it. We fully understood that what we were being told to do was very important for Joan's well being. There were no options other than going ahead with all the treatments. We knew Joan had to have these tests and procedures to get all better. After many tests and procedures, she was ready for the operation to remove the tumor that was cancerous. [4/14/03] After the operation, she had many more tests to get her ready for the treatments to make sure that the cancer was gone and would not come back. As we have stated, the treatments were chemo for four months and radiation for one and a half months, also during these treatments there would be many tests to see how Joan was handling everything. If it were not for the quality of Doctor's and nurses that Joan had and is still having, I don 't think we could have gotten as far as we have come which is to the end of the chemo treatment. I really mean it. The decision to go with the Doctors that we chose was the best decision that we could have made and we thank God for helping us to make that decision. The nurses came along with the Doctors and they were also the very best. As far as our emotions go and how we handled everything to this point I'd have to say that without the support of our family and friends and of course without God and all the prayers it could have been a very different outcome. We, at this point, are OK and are gearing ourselves up for the next procedure which is the radiation treatments. Going through this illness is a very stressful thing to do. At times we find ourselves getting irritable with each other. This is I guess normal because we get so tired from being so busy that the frustration has to come out somewhere. We do a lot of counting to ten

maybe two or three times in a row. One thing we do is never go to sleep at night without a hug and a kiss and an "I love you." This is important because you always have another day to start on when you wake up. If you get up mad at one another you will never make it through the day. We will be married fifty one years this October 26th and we certainly must have done something right not only to have stayed together but to still be in LOVE, like we were only married yesterday. [Well almost.] A few things might have changed but I think that comes with age? It is very important that you don't dwell on the bad things that happen. You must think positive and think about how good it is going to be when everything is OK again. All in all I think everything went as well as could be expected. I am kind of proud of both of us for hanging in there. [PS - A side effect of chemo is being very, very tired all the time. I can surely attest to that. Joan was super tired every day and she still is. You do sort of get used to it and find ways to work around it.]

September 20, 2003

We woke up on the early side this morning because Lewis was coming to work on the yard. I needed to be out there with him at the start to tell him exactly what we wanted done. One of our low palm trees died and we had to rearrange everything after he took it out in the front yard. Everything came out OK and now we just have to put in a tree to take the place of the palm that died. We decided to replace it with a Florida Gardenia tree which will look real good and have a real nice scent. Joan felt pretty good today - no nausea and her body not to achy. After we had our breakfast we were going to try and go to the mall, we need a new toaster and thought the outing would do us both good. We did a few things around the house that took us longer than we expected and the time just slid right on by to a point that it would have been to late to go to the mall. We decided not to push ourselves and plan the trip to the mall for tomorrow. It seems that we can only do one thing in a day or Joan will get to tired, we should know that by now. Oh well, like they say there's always tomorrow. I think the Mall will still be there on Sunday. We did not eat lunch until late so we mixed dinner with lunch and called it a day as far as eating goes. That of course does not include a late snack maybe around nine thirty. As Joan says, it must be time for an ice cream soda. I think today is just about over for us so I will say goodnight. Goodnight.

September 21, 2003

We awoke, had breakfast, took a shower and decided not to do anything until it was time to go to the mall. We hung around until two thirty and then decided to leave for the mall. We wanted to buy a new toaster, some wine glasses and a decanter to put the wine in. We also wanted to buy a bath mat so Joan would not slip and fall while taking a shower. Joan never took showers until recently. She takes showers now so she can do her hair, or what's ever up there. She does not really have anything to really speak of but it makes her happy to wash it anyway - why not. The hair is really starting to make a break-through in spots but will take a while before you can say I just washed my hair.

After we finished shopping, we stopped at our Daughter Kim's house to pay her a surprise visit. Kim and the whole family were really surprised to see us, I guess it has been at least one and a half months since we went to Kim's, ever since Joan's immune system broke down. We had a great visit with Kim and all the kids. After our visit with Kim we went to Friendless for dinner and of course some ice cream, and then home. We were tired from our very long overdue outing, so we got ready for bed and watched the Emmy's, until it was time to go to sleep. I better say goodnight now. Goodnight.

September 22, 2003

We are up and feeling pretty good. Joan has no nausea but is very tired. After yesterday I kind of expected her to be. Yesterday was such a nice day, especially the part where we visited Kim and the kids. Today will most likely be a rest up day for Joan. I need to do a few things outside. We received a phone call from Laura Johnson this morning telling us that she was in Florida and only about two hours away from us. Laura is just like family to us, so needles to say we were real happy with the thought of seeing her. We made arrangements to have them come to our house on Tuesday about noon time for a couple of days or for as long as she wants. Joan is up for the visit even though she is tired. We have not seen Laura for a long time and have a lot to catch up on. Laura lived in Park Ridge, NJ. Also, they were our neighbors at the Jersey Shore, in Normandy Shores. Joan after lunch had a nap for at least two hours, while I was outside doing my thing with the yard. We were going to have dinner about six o'clock – steak, baked potato, tomato and corn on the cob with cherry pie for dessert. sounds good and was good. After dinner we did what we usually do - t/v, bed and go to sleep. See you all in the AM. Goodnight.

September 23, 24, 25, and 26, 2003

I put these four days together seeing that Laura and John were visiting. Laura and John arrived about 1:30 PM on Tuesday. It was real good to see Laura whom we have not seen for at least one and a half years. John we did not know until Laura introduced us to him. After they got settled into our guest room, we just sat around and chatted to bring us up to date with everything Laura has been doing and everything that we have been doing. After talking for about three hours we decided to go out for dinner and talk some more. We went to the Manor at the PGA Village. It was nice and not too busy so we really enjoyed ourselves. After dinner we came right home because Joan was tired and needed to lie down. I think it was about 10:30 PM when we all decided that it was time to call it a day and go to bed. Joan handled the day quite well, no nausea but extremely tired. Laura knew how sick Joan has been from our phone conversations with her in NJ. I'm sure that is what prompted her to make a visit with Joan.

Wednesday we all got up about 9:00 AM and had a real good breakfast; eggs, Taylor ham and English muffins toasted with butter and some fruit and coffee.

After breakfast, Laura and Joan continued to talk about old times, about the kids and what they were doing. John and I went outside to look at our garden. Joan still holding up pretty well, but you could tell that she was getting tired and needed a rest. Joan rested for a couple of hours and the rest of us just hung out and took it easy. Laura and John wanted to get on the internet to see if they had any E-mail on their computer in NJ. About 4:00 PM we all went to look at our PGA condo and show them all the good things that were at the PGA. After leaving the PGA, we went out to eat at a very nice restaurant on Rt. 1 in Port St Lucie. We had a real good time. Joan again needed to go home because she got real tired, but we were real proud of her for holding up as well as she has been doing. After we got home we all decided to call it a day so we went to bed and that was that for Wednesday.

Thursday morning was the day John and I plaid golf. It was the first time that I plaid golf since Joan got sick and it was the first time that John had plaid in two years. We had a great time. Laura stayed at home with Joan. After golf Laura and John took a trip to Deerfield, which is South of us. Joan and I had to go to the Doctor's in Stuart to get Joan's blood checked and to see how the white and red blood cells were behaving. Joan's white cell count was right on target and so was her immune system, not so with the red blood cells, they were very low which meant that she was still anemic. The Doctor gave Joan medicine to help produce more red blood cells and also gave her iron which helps the red blood cell count. Joan needs to have all her blood counts to be normal before she starts the radiation procedure. If it does not get normal soon, she will have to have a blood transfusion which we are not too happy about. We arrived home about 5:30 PM. We had dinner and by then Joan was about done in. When Joan goes for her blood check ups she usually gets real tired and all she wants to do is go to bed - which she did, right after we had dinner. We did not expect Laura and John to come back from there little trip until about 10:30 PM. I waited for them and Joan went to sleep. After they got home we talked for a little while until we all got so tired that we all decided to go to bed. Laura told me they would be leaving about noon tomorrow so we all said goodnight.

Friday morning we all got up about 8:00 AM, all except Joan. She stayed in bed until about 9:30 AM. We all had breakfast and just sat around and talked until about 11:30 AM. I guess it was time that Laura and John got ready to go, they packed their car and we said our good-byes. We all felt a bit sad, but we all knew we would be seeing each other soon again.

Laura wants to stay at our condo in March for a month with her Daughter Evie and her husband. Joan and I love Evie very much so it will be something to look forward to. After Laura and John left, Joan and I took it easy for the rest of the day. Joan was very tired and to be perfectly honest so was I. We had supper about 7:30 PM and then just decided to go to bed and [here we go again] watch T/V until we fell asleep. I'd better say goodnight now. Goodnight.

September 27, 2003

Today we got up about 9:00 AM, had breakfast and just lingered around the breakfast table reading the paper. Joan did not feel real great. She felt kind of nauseous for some reason. We both felt a little depressed, maybe because Laura and John were not here. It was rather nice having company to talk to. It sort of took our minds off the problems we have. Oh well, we will get back in the swing of things real quick I'm sure. We really did not do anything today except take it easy. I was a little busy outside with Lewis and Rocky the gardeners just watching what they were doing. Our yard is really getting quite nice and is very nice to look at. The way Joan is feeling today we decided to go very easy with what we had to eat. Breakfast was the regular, lunch was half a sandwich each and dinner was soup and a glass of milk for me and water for Joan. We watched some T/V and turned in early, that's getting to be a way of life for us. Goodnight.

September 28, 2003

Joan still not feeling to good, she woke up feeling nauseous and her legs are hurting from the knees down. The nausea could still be from the chemo but I do not think the legs have anything to do with the cancer problem, unless it is because she was so inactive, and now that she is moving around more they are feeling the strain. I guess we will just have to wait and see how they do. My heart really goes out to Joan when I see how upset she is getting with feeling sick all the time. It is going on eight months that she has been feeling sick and just not herself. There has been a day here and there that she was feeling good but that is not nearly enough to keep her spirits up. We knew from the git-go that it was not going to be a cake walk, so we will just have to think more positive and count on all the prayers a bit more and I'm sure everything will turn out OK. We go to Doctor Griffis on Monday, the 29th for what reason I'm not sure so I will call him in the morning to find out. I'm sure it is not to start the radiation and we know that Joan's blood levels are not right yet to start the radiation. We will see what he says in the morning. We did not see anyone today, but we did talk to almost everyone on the phone.

Our neighbors across the street are moving and are having the closing on their house on the ninth of October which means they must be out of the house that day. They seem to have a problem because Fred needs to have an operation which will keep them here for at least another month [sorry there names are Joann and Fred]. Joann called us to find out if they could rent our PGA Condo until Fred is better. I will take them to the condo to show them what it looks like and if they would like to rent it. I'm sure they will like it so it just might work out very nice for them. The Condo is only two to three minutes away from here so it would be very convenient for them. It would be nice if we could help them and it just might take our minds off what is going on with us. The rest of our day was very quiet. We watched a couple of videos which were better than the shows on T/V. We need to do that more often. We skipped over dinner. Neither Joan nor I felt up to eating anything. We had a late lunch and were not at all hungry. I think we will close for today. Talk to you tomorrow. Goodnight.

September 29, 2003

Today I was awakened by a phone call from Martin Memorial billing department at 8:30 AM. They goofed on some billing and needed to ask me some questions about what insurance we had. They have had all the records for some time now so it must have been an error in the computer. It sure is funny if I call them at 8:30 AM, I get "Our office hours are from 9:30 AM to 4:00 PM." If they call me, time is not an issue. My office must be open 24 hours a day - so they must think. OH, WELL.

Joan was very restless last night, her legs were hurting badly. I rubbed them down with the pain relief at least three times and each time I did, it only gave her some relief for a short time. We are going to find out what is going on with her legs, it seems to be getting worse. The Doctor's so far have not been able to come up with a solution to make her legs better. Since Joan has not been on the chemo treatment, the legs have been worse. It seems that we just go from one problem to another. Today was not a good day. Joan was in bed all day because of her legs so I had to call Doctor Griffis' office and cancel Joan's appointment for today. Doctor Griffis told me that they were only going to take some pictures and that they could do that when we came in next Friday. The rest of the day was spent trying to make Joan comfortable. I did the best I could but it didn't seem to be to helpful. Joan slept a lot which was good. While sleeping she did not hurt. We finished the day as usual and prayed that tomorrow will be better.

Goodnight.

September 30, 2003

Joan woke me up about 7:00 AM this morning with a lot of pain in her legs. I guess we had been up two or three times last night with Joan's legs hurting. We did not go back to sleep, we just took care of Joan's legs the best we could. Carol came to clean today, the house needed it after having company for about four days. The company did not get the house dirty they are very tidy people, the reason it got dirty is that the house had some activity in it. When Joan and I are home alone we practically live in the bedroom with Joan feeling the way she does. I called Doctor Iannotti to have Joan's prescription for pain pills refilled. Without them Joan does not do well. Again the leg problem is really not connected with the cancer problem. It is just a shame that Joan has to have both of these problems at the same time, it sure does not give us a break at all. Joan has not felt nauseous since the other day. Thank you God.

We do not have any Doctor appointments for Joan until Friday, so we thought we could get a good rest without going all the time. Some day I'm sure we will get back to a normal way of life. We ate fairly well today - breakfast was our normal breakfast; lunch was bacon and tomato sandwiches [very good]; dinner was vegetable soup for Joan and I had poached eggs on English muffins a real favorite of mine [I know it sounds like breakfast but I like it any time]. It seems like things are going real bad for us but really it probably is the way it has to be until we are all done with the procedures that will get rid of the cancer that Joan had. I can't say that it hasn't been tough because it has been, but at the same time it will not be forever and we will get our life back. We know we can get through it and we know we will. It will most likely be a year before we can get some normalcy back into our life's but the good part is that Joan will have a life to get back to, and that is what makes this all worth while. Our Doctors, as I said before, have been just great. They are not only excellent doctors and the best in their field, but they are real good human beings that are real concerned with getting their patients all healthy again. We are real fortunate in having them, believe me. I think it is time to say goodnight. Goodnight.

Voice of the Children

Did it ever occur to you she might die?

I never thought about her dying, even though my best friend died from breast cancer. For some reason I just never thought about it. All I thought about was her getting better. I think in my Heart I knew she would be OK. *Diane*

I never even thought that this would be so severe that she would die. Like I said before my parents have gone thru so many health problems they have always made it through. We all are very fortunate that we have God on our side to help us. *Kim*

I don't think I ever considered that. Either I was in denial or just ignorant of the severity of the disease. The few people I have known throughout my life that had breast cancer (including my mom's mom) recovered from it. I was a little more shook up after the surgery when we found out that they had to remove more than they expected. *Ken*

My mother dying in my mind was not an option. I have a strong faith as so does my father and we both had many conversations with God praying to keep them both strong and safe. In the same way that a child needs a parent giving them the confidence and reassurance to learn to walk and talk to grow and face adversities, we need to look to our faith in God. That he will absolutely pick us up when we fall, carry us through the hard times and teach us to do the same time and time again. Without our faith there would be no hope and hope is what we need to survive. The two work hand and hand. The battle is won but the fight is not over. Both of my parents are aging, something I cannot change. Their health is strained in many different ways, not just with the cancer, which Thank God we believe to be gone. So there is still a lot of caring and support that needs to be given, something they never kept from me. So without hesitation I will do what needs to be done love them with all my heart and pray that I can be just like them, loving and caring and strong enough to make it through. *Doreen*

October

October 1, 2003

Today we woke up at 7:00 AM. Joan had an appointment with Doctor Kass, Joan's Neurologist, concerning Joan's legs and the pain that she is having with them. We arrived at Doctor Kass' office at 9:30 AM and signed in. Doctor Kass examined Joan and could really not find any real reason for all the pain Joan is having in her legs. The doctor said she has a small amount of Neuropathy but not enough to give Joan the pain that she is experiencing. Doctor Kass told Joan that she should go to a pain specialist to find out just where the pain is coming from. She gave us a Doctor's name to see, and also told us to discuss this problem with Doctor Iannotti so it would not interfere with what he is doing with the medicines he is giving to Joan. We will talk to Doctor Iannotti on Friday. Also, we will talk to Doctor Griffis when we see him on Friday. Joan is feeling a little better since she now is taking the pain medicine again. After we left Doctor Kass's office we went straight home. We had lunch and Joan went to lie down for a rest. I had to go to the PGA Condo to check on a few things that needed to be done. No matter how you might feel, life still goes on and things still need to be done. I finished what I had to do at the Condo and went right home. I am super tired today so I think I might lie down and take a rest also. We had dinner and thought we might watch another video instead of the T/V. Will talk to you tomorrow Goodnight - PS – Before Joan went to bed she did feel a little nauseous. This is pretty normal just before she goes to see Doctor Iannotti which she will do on Friday. Its not the Doctor that makes her nauseous it's the idea of the treatment she needs to take. Goodnight, again.

October 2, 2003

We did not have to get up early today so we didn't. It really felt good to just lie in bed for as long as we wanted too. I think we got out of bed about 10:30 AM, had breakfast, took a shower and got dressed for the day. Joan for some reason felt a little nauseous today but really not to bad. Joan usually gets a little nervous when she knows she is going to seethe Doctor. It's a little nerve racking when she knows the Doctor is going to let her know weather she will need a blood transfusion or not. We go tomorrow for blood work and for the Iron shot which is given intravenously. The blood work will tell weather Joan needs a blood transfusion or not. We pray that she will not need one. I went to the Motor Vehicle to get our new registration for the Benz., which has to be renewed by the 5th of Oct. We are now good for another year. Joan is still a little nauseous so we just hung around the house and did much of nothing the rest of the day. I am really very tired so it is probably good I do not have to do too much. We will have dinner and most likely - yep, watch some T/V and go to bed. Say goodnight Ken. Goodnight.

October 3, 2003

It is 8:30 AM and we are up and at 'em. I guess we had enough sleep and have decided to stay up and start the day. We will have breakfast, take a shower, get dressed and get ready to go to the Doctor's. We need to go to both Doctors today. First to Doctor Griffis and then to Doctor Iannotti. Doctor Griffis needs to take a couple of pictures of Joan for the radiation procedure, he also needs to know from Doctor Iannotti if Joan's blood counts are OK or whether she will need a blood transfusion before he starts the radiation treatment. After we left Doctor Griffis's office we went right upstairs to our other appointment with Doctor Iannotti to have the blood work done and also the iron shot to be given to Joan. Thank God the red cell count was OK. Doctor Iannotti said we will not have to have a blood transfusion and that we can start the radiation treatment as soon as Doctor Griffis says OK. We are really very glad that we can now get on with the rest of Joan's treatments. It seems that we were stalled out for a while but are now ready to go. We went right downstairs to Doctor Griffis's office to give him the sheet with all the blood counts on it. This is what he was waiting for, so his nurse made our first radiation treatment for next Monday at 12:00 PM. It looks like that will be what we will be doing for the next six weeks every day except Saturday and Sunday. OH WELL, we have to get it over with, so lets do it. After we left the Doctor's offices we decided to get dinner at the Ale House. Clams on the half shell with a nice cold root beer for me and two hamburgers each with a root beer for Joan. The hamburgers are small ones and are very good. French fries and salad also go with it. After eating we went right home and made some phone calls to all our kids who were waiting to hear about what happened at the Doctor's. Joan did not do too bad with dinner seeing that she was a little nauseous to start with. After calling all the kids we hung it up for the night and went to bed, T/V and to sleep. Goodnight.

October 4 & 5, 2003

Saturday and Sunday were two days just about the same, except Sunday the fifth was my birthday. Saturday we just hung out around the house doing whatever needed to be done and we also talked a lot about what the Doctors had to say on Friday, concerning Joan's blood levels and the starting of the radiation treatment, which starts on Monday, the sixth of October. Everything is A-OK for the radiation treatment. The blood levels are good enough to start, so the Doctors say. Joan, on the other hand is not completely sure she feels up to it at this time. We had a long discussion about it and came to the conclusion that Joan was just nervous about start-ing. I really thought she was up to it and it was time we got the program started. It is going to be a lengthy program so we need to get started now. If we wait too long it might not be to good for what has already been done.

Sunday - My birthday - Well I guess it is just another day. I do not feel my age so I thought I would start counting backward. I don't think that will help because I feel a lot older than I am. When you get middle aged like I am and you feel older, you might as well tell the truth. I really am not middle aged it is more like the high middle age. Oh Ok, I'm seventy six years old and I don't feel a day older then ninety six. We really did not do to much today, until dinner which we had at Bob Evan's Restaurant. After dinner we went to our Daughter Kim's house for birthday cake and coffee. It was special to see everyone at Kim's. It gave us a chance to see how the addition on the house was coming along. The first floor is all framed out and looks real good. Joan felt pretty good today as far as the nausea goes. Being tired is a whole other story. When we got home at 9:30 PM, Joan about fell into bed, and was asleep no later than 10:00 PM. I watched a little T/V, sports, and fell asleep while doing so.

Radiation: Day One (First Week)

October 6, 2003

I woke up at 6:30 AM so I could get a shower and dressed before I woke Joan up. Today we start the radiation treatment and have to leave at 11:00 AM so we are there by 12:00 PM. We actually got there at 11:45 and they took Joan right away. I settled down in the waiting room for what I thought would be at least an hour, when all of a sudden Joan came into the waiting room and said let's go, I'm all done. The whole treatment took only one half hour and we were on our way. Joan said it was really OK and was not even uncomfortable, maybe a little warm feeling , but really OK. We left home at eleven and were back home by one. If we could do that every time we go, it won't be to bad.

When we got home we had lunch. After lunch Joan decided to take a nap. She was very tired. I think Joan had worked herself up over the thought that the radiation was going to be a hard thing to do, but it was really a very pleasant surprise that it was not. I think that the hardest thing about the radiation program was the map and the tattoos that they had to put on Joan's upper body. It took a while to do and was kind of uncomfortable for Joan to lie in the position that she had to be in. Joan also did not know whether it would hurt and that worried her. We were told that it would not hurt but you know how the mind works. I guess you need to find out for yourself. Joan can not stand pain. Her tolerance for pain is Zero. I guess the only other hard thing about the radiation treatment is the amount of time it is going to take to complete the program; every day for six weeks, but we will get through it and Joan is going to be just fine. I might need a little help when it is finished just taking the steering wheel out of my hands. Just kidding I can stand anything as long as I know it is going to help Joan. I really think that the hardest part of Joan's program is getting to feel that the cancer is behind us. It is still a long haul before we will be all done, and she still has a lot of testing to go through just to make sure that she is cancer free, but I do think that the hardest part is over.

After Joan's nap it was about time for dinner. Boy, does the time fly when you're having fun. Dinner is over. We made a few calls and now it is time to turn in, you know what that means. You got it - T/V and to sleep. Goodnight.

Radiation: Day Two

October 7, 2003

Up at 7:30 this morning. I got myself all ready for the day and then I woke Joan up. I guess that was about 8:30. Joan was quite tired but got right up and got ready for the day. Today was Joan's second day for the radiation treatment, we thought we would leave at 11:00 AM, the same as yesterday and see how we do today. We had breakfast and got ready to go. We left the house exactly at 11:00 AM. We were at the Doctor's office at 11:45. Again, they took Joan right in for her treatment. It seems that I no sooner sat down in the waiting room than Joan was out and ready to go home. I guess it took about twenty minutes; about the same as yesterday. Joan said every thing went real good - just like the first treatment. Joan was very happy about how things were going and we hope it will continue this way for all the remaining treatments.

Joan, outside of being tired, felt pretty good this morning - no nausea and very little aches. We arrived home from the Doctor's office at 12:30, which is fantastic. That means the whole procedure took one and one half hours, starting from our house to the Doctor's office, having the treatment and returning back to our house. Not bad. As soon as we got in the house we decided to have lunch before Joan got too tired to eat. Me too. Getting up early is going to change how we do things. We eat earlier so we get hungry sooner for lunch, which means we will probably want to have dinner earlier. I think that is the way it is supposed to be. After lunch Joan did go for the nap. When Joan say's she is going to take a nap, that means she is going to bed for a sleep. She means business - under the covers and all.

I did some paper work, and checked out my Christmas decorations, Debbie was coming over about six tonight to see what she is going to do for all the Christmas decorations this year. Debbie is a decorator and has been doing our decorations ever since we moved here. She is a delight and we would not know what to do with out her.

Dinner tonight was a big nothing, neither Joan or I felt like eating at all. We had a good breakfast and a good lunch so we skipped dinner. I'm sure we will snack on something before we go to bed, which I'm sure will be very early. So I think I will say goodnight now. See you all tomorrow.

PS: THIS WAS A GOOD DAY.

Radiation: Day Three

October 8, 2003

Joan and I both got up at 8:00 AM this morning, a little later than yes-terday. We showered, got dressed and had breakfast all by 10:00 AM. Joan for some reason did not feel to good this morning - that old nauseous feel-ing again. Joan has not really felt nauseous for about five days, so we really do not know where this is coming from. It should not be coming from the radiation and we thought the nausea from the chemo would be all gone by now, maybe not. Joan says it feels the same as the nausea she had from the chemo. We will wait and see how she feels later after the radiation is done for today. We left for the Doctor's office at 11:00 AM, the same as yesterday. We arrived at the Doctor's office at 11:45 - again the same as yesterday. They took Joan right away. Joan was out in the waiting room all set to go home by 12:05 and that was with them taking two extra pictures beside the radiation. The time it takes seems to be getting shorter each day. We arrived home about 12:40 PM which is also very good time. When we arrived home Joan still did not feel to good. She still had the nauseous feel-ing. It was about time for lunch and the only thing that sounded good to Joan was soup. So, I made her some vegetable soup and she ate it all. I had a sandwich and a glass of milk. Joan was pretty tired and about ready to take a nap, so that is what she did. While Joan was sleeping, I did some paper work and tried hard to keep my eye's open, I guess the getting up early has gotten to me, so I laid down on the coach and I guess I fell sound asleep. The next thing I felt was Joan shaking me and telling me it was about 4:30 PM. I must have slept for a couple of hours or more. I have to go to a Granada Isle board meeting at 7:00 PM tonight and we still need to have dinner. I decided to go to KFC and bring home some fried chicken, mashed potato's and some coleslaw. We like that every now and than. By the time we finished dinner it was time for me to go to the meeting. The meeting was about two hours long, but it was a good meeting. Afterwards, I went right home, changed into my pajamas and headed for bed. Joan was already there and to my surprise was still awake. We watched a little T/V and then we decided to go to sleep. Goodnight. PS - Joan felt a little better and the nausea seems to have gone.

Radiation: Day Four

October 9, 2003

Today we have to go to Doctor Iannotti's office before we go to Doctor Griffis's office for the radiation. We need to have Joan's blood checked and she also needs an iron shot intravenously, After checking Joan's blood levels Doctor Iannotti said that Joan needed a shot to build up her immune system which went low again. I guess they sort of thought this would happen due to the radiation. [Another side effect to deal with; OH, WELL] We left for the Doctor's at 10:30 AM and arrived there at 11:15 AM. We went right up to Iannotti's office for our 11:15 AM appointment. We then went downstairs to Doctor Griffis's office for the radiation appointment at 12:00 PM. They took Joan right away. The first thing they did to Joan was to take more pictures. [I need to find out why.] After the pictures they started the radiation treatment which only took about fifteen minutes. Joan was in the waiting room to get me no later than 12:20 PM We left and arrived home at a little after 1:00 PM. Not too bad, all in all. We left home at 10:30 AM and were back home at 1:00 PM. That is a total of two and a half hours for everything we had to do. After arriving home we had lunch and, of course, Joan thought she would take a little nap. It really is tiring for Joan, both physically and mentally. I had some things around the house to do but I also might take a short nap. When they said that the only side effect that the radiology would have was getting very tired, they were not kidding. Joan is even more tired now than when she was going through chemo. Joan told me that they took more pictures today as they had yesterday. We did not know why, so I thought I had better call the Doctor's office and find out. At first we thought they might be looking for something and of course you always think the worst. I did call and spoke to the nurse that was doing the procedure and she told me that they had to see if any of the tattoos had moved, caused by any swelling that could occur. This of course put us at ease and made us feel much better. I guess we shouldn't second guess what they are doing. They are pretty good at telling us what is going on but I guess this one slid by. After Joan woke up from her nap, we had dinner and just talked about what I had found out. I did not take a nap like I thought I would so I am the one now who is super tired. I guess we will turn in early tonight so we can get up on time for tomorrows trip to the Doctors. Tomorrow will be the last procedure of the first week so we can look forward to the two days, Saturday and Sunday, off. I think I will sign off now, so I will say goodnight. Goodnight.

Radiation: Day Five

October 10, 2003

Today is the last day of the first week of our radiation program. We have, I believe, five more weeks to go. Tomorrow and the next day we do not have any radiation treatments or Doctor appointments to go to. It is like we will be on vacation with nothing to do. I think we will catch up on our sleep. We have been getting up early this whole week to make sure we make our appointments on time. The problem is that we do not go to bed any earlier than we always did. This morning we left for the Doctor's office at 11:00 AM and returned home at 12:30 PM. I think that is real good time. Joan was not really feeling too good. She has that nausea feeling again. It must be that the chemo is not all out of her system yet, and the medicine she is taking to increase her blood levels might be causing the nausea also. The nausea is not as bad as it was but is still very annoying. The first week of radiation was not to bad. In fact it could not have gone any better compared with what we thought it would be like. The trip to Stuart every day went rather well. The traffic was not a problem. I guess we were leaving just at the right time and coming home at the right time to miss the bad traffic times. Outside of Joan feeling a little nauseous and very tired, there were no other medical problems to speak of. Joan woke up from her nap late in the afternoon - about the time we start thinking of what to have for dinner. We made it easy tonight. We ordered Chinese and it was good. They opened up a new Chinese restaurant very close by. Actually it has been a Chinese restaurant and some one new took it over. The new owners are very nice and improved on the food that they serve. It really is very good. After dinner we just talked for a while and kind of thought about what we will do for the next couple of days, seeing that we are on "vacation". We got as far as let's sleep late and figure it all out when we get up. Joan feels a little better, but very tired again. I'm tired also so I think we will go to bed, watch T/V and go to sleep. Goodnight.

October 11 & 12, 2003

These two days are our "vacation" days since we do not have to go to chemo, radiation or any Doctor's or procedures for forty eight hours. Saturday we got up about 9:30 AM and did not have to get ready to go anywhere. We had a nice leisurely breakfast and read the paper without having to rush. The rest of the day Joan rested and watched T/V. I worked on my computer for about three hours and got myself real frustrated. My computer and printer are not in sync with one another so I can't print anything that I write. After trying to fix the problem for the three hours, I decided it would be better to call Circuit City and find out if they have a service department that could fix it for me. I talked to a salesman and he said that I could buy a new one and most likely a more up to date one for a lot less then it would cost to fix the one I have. I think he is right so I am going to go there on Monday after Joan's radiation treatment and look at what they have. Joan had a small amount of the nausea feeling today but not too bad. I, of course, had a headache from the computer. Other than that, we felt pretty good. We skipped lunch today - we were really not hungry. We had dinner kind of late, somewhere around 7:30 PM. After we ate dinner we just took it easy until bed time. Sunday, we got up a little on the late side, 10:30 AM to be exact. We ate breakfast and I guess the rest of the day was very similar to Saturday. Joan did not seem to have any nausea, which of course was great. We both were tired and were enjoying not having to go anyplace, especially to the Doctor's or for any treatments. We will most likely watch golf and the baseball playoffs. Feels good to do just what we are doing. I think for some reason we both feel a little more relaxed about our situation. It kind of feels like we are in the last innings and have the feeling that we are winning. We hope and pray that this feeling will continue until Joan is all better. We again skipped lunch [not hungry again] but will have a good dinner, most likely about the same time as yesterday. I think I will close for today. It looks like the rest of the day will be dinner and watch T/V and go to bed. If it turns out to be anything else and interesting I will tell you tomorrow. Goodnight. PS. It was nice two have the two day s off from running.

Radiation: Day Six (Second Week)

October 13, 2003

Today is the first day of the second week of the radiation treatment. We got up at 7:30 AM, took a shower, got dressed and had our breakfast. Does that sound familiar or what? Joan feels pretty good. So far, no nausea but as usual very tired and achy legs. After breakfast we hung out for a little while until it was time to leave for the Doctor's to get the radiation treatment. We left at 11:00 AM and arrived at the Doctor's office at 11:35 AM - not bad. Joan had to wait about ten minutes before they took her. That is the first time they did not take her right away. I guess it was because we were so early and we really are not the only patient they have. It just seems that way - only kidding. When we left the Doctor's office we went right home. We had the A/C man coming at 2:00 PM to service our A/C unit. Our electric bills have been running rather high for the last couple of months and we felt that the A/C has been the problem.

It turned out to be the right assumption, because there was definitely a problem with the A/C that caused it to run more than it should. We had it fixed and will wait to see if that was the problem when we get our next bill. Enough of that, we will get back to getting Joan fixed again. I think Joan slept the whole time the A/C man was here - about two hours or so.

I had some things to do in the office and I also wanted to watch what the A/C man was doing, After the A/C man left it was time for dinner. Tonight we felt like some soup, so that is what we had. I know Joan is going to want a snack later. I wonder what she will have. Maybe an ice cream soda or an ice cream. I think I'm losing it. [I really know that is what she is going to have, she has one almost every night].

I think I will watch a little baseball tonight. I haven't kept up with what is going on, so I guess it is time I catch up. Joan still feels pretty good as far as the nausea goes, so at least she feels more comfortable. I will talk to you all tomorrow OK. Goodnight. PS. We originally thought that the nausea would stop after chemo, so maybe that is what is happening now - hope so.

Radiation: Day Seven

October 14, 2003

Up at 8:00 AM - a little later than yesterday, but not to bad. We got ready for the day, had breakfast and just hung around until it was time to leave for the Doctor's. We left as usual at 11:00 AM and arrived at the Doctor's office at 11:45 AM. They took Joan right away. They took more pictures and gave her the radiation treatment that she was to have We left the Doctor's office at 12:10 PM and went right home, arriving at 12:45 PM. We have been doing just great time-wise since we started the radiation program. Joan feels OK today - no nausea and not quite as tired as she was yesterday. Joan's sinuses bother her today but she can handle that with no problem. [It say's here.] We ate lunch and just sat around and talked, mostly about how Joan was doing and how we thought she was feeling compared to how she felt a week ago. I thought that there was a significant improvement and Joan thought that she was doing a little better. My judgement was based on how she was acting and how she looked. Joan seemed to have more pep and was starting to do a few things around the house that she was not at all interested in doing before. Her face does not look as drawn as it was. I believe Joan thinks she is doing better but she has been there before and then all of a sudden she would feel awful again. Maybe she is just going to wait a little while longer before passing judgement on her progress. After all it is her body and she should know better then anyone how she is doing. After our discussion I sat in my chair and for some reason fell asleep for about two and a half hours. It is time to start thinking about dinner, well almost. Joan also fell asleep in the bedroom. Tonight our daughter Kim and Sierra came to visit while Sammy was at soccer practice. We had a real good time, it is always a pleasure for us to see our daughter and grandchildren. [We did eat dinner before Kim came]. After Kim left we got in our pajamas and settled in for the night. There was not too much on the T/V, so we watched a little news and decided to go to sleep. Goodnight.

Radiation: Day Eight

October 15, 2003

    This morning we got up at 8:00AM, got ready for the day, had breakfast and left for the Doctor's at 11:00 AM. We arrived at the Doctor's at 11:30 AM. Boy, did we ever make time this morning. There were hardly any cars on the road so the trip was a good one. Joan seems to be OK today. She says she does not feel nauseous at all and we hope it stays that way. She is of course still very tired but is trying real hard to do a few things after we leave the Doctor's. Today on our way home we stopped at Circuit City to look at a new printer for my computer. We made one more stop before going home and that was to go to the fruit store and of course, we bought some fruit. By now Joan was on all fours. When we returned home we had a quick lunch, Joan had remembered that she was to be at her nail salon to have her nails done at 2:00 PM . Joan would not miss her nail appointment even if she had to crawl there. We made the appointment by the skin of our teeth. I think it was about two minutes after two when we got there. When we left the nail salon Joan was very shaky [as she calls it]. I think we over did it which we will not do again. Of that you can be sure. Joan was really very tired. I am very proud of Joan for wanting to do some things, but we have to space them out a little better. We have a long way to go with the radiation, so if we did one thing after her treatment every other day that would be fine I'm sure. When we finally got home, all Joan wanted to do was to lie down and that is what she did. Joan rested until it was dinner time. After we had dinner Joan went to bed to watch T/V until it was time to go to sleep. I believe after I go to the store, I will be doing the same thing, so I will say goodnight now. Goodnight.

Radiation: Day Nine

October 16, 2003

    Up and at 'em at 7:00 AM this morning. We need an early start today because we have to be at the Doctor's office at 11:15 AM. [Doctor Iannotti first] And then on to Doctor Griffis' office by 12:00 PM. Joan needs her blood checked and then go to her radiation treatment. We are all excited and happy with the results of Joan's blood levels from the test that she just had taken. Doctor Iannotti told us that she is no longer a anemic and would not need any more Iron shots,. In fact, Joan would not need any more of any kind of shots. Her blood levels are all normal, thank God. Doctor Iannotti said he would see us when Joan is all done with her radiation program unless we need him for any reason. Doctor Iannotti was pleased with everything and said that Joan really had a very hard time with everything and it was time that she had some good news. Doctor Griffis also was pleased with the blood levels and will be in touch with us concerning Joan having a flu shot. After we left Doctor Griffis's office we went right home for lunch and for Joan to take it easy. [We don't want to duplicate yesterday.] After Joan's rest we might go out for dinner - nothing big just a local restaurant and come right home again. We need to call all the kids tonight to tell them the good news we got from the tests today. Well it is 5:00PM and Joan said she feels up to going out to eat dinner, so off we went, to a nice Italian restaurant on Rt. # 1. It's only about fifteen minutes from home. We had a nice dinner and just relaxed for a while. When we finished dinner we went right home. Joan did not waste any time getting ready for bed. I listened to our message machine to see what messages there where if any. Yep, there were three messages, one from Doctor Griffis' office telling us that Joan could now have a flu shot. The second message was from Doreen so I got a chance to tell her the good news about her Mom. She was real pleased. The third message was from the A/C man, nothing important. I called all the other kids and told them what the Doctors said today. They were all very happy and felt very positive about the outcome of their Mom's condition. [Me too.] I think I will watch baseball again tonight and then turn in for the night. We can sleep a little longer in the morning because we only have one Doctor appointment for the day. I think I will say goodnight now, but will talk to you tomorrow. Goodnight.

Radiation: Day Ten

October 17, 2003

We got up at 7:30 AM. We are back on the regular schedule as far as getting up is concerned. We showered, shaved, [I shaved, not Joan], had breakfast and relaxed until it was time to leave for the Doctor's. It took us thirty five Mounties to get to the Doctor's - no traffic again. [After we had breakfast we did get dressed before we left for the Doctor's.] The times we have been leaving are just right, we get the minimum of traffic which makes the trip more enjoyable. Joan has had no trouble with the radiation treatment, no swelling and no blemishes on the areas that they treat. I am so happy that she is doing as well as she is with the radiation. She had so much trouble with the chemo and the blood levels that it's time she got a break. On our way home we stopped at Circuit City and bought a new printer for my computer. When we left Circuit City we went right home and had some lunch. After lunch, Joan took a rest and I worked on setting up my computer. I worked on it for at least two hours or more only to find out that the new printer was not compatible with the old computer. Oh well, that will be a whole new story that I will save for another time. Joan woke up about 4:30 PM, so I decided to start dinner which was lamb chops, corn on the cob and a baked potato. Um Um - Joan has been eating a little better. I think it is because she feels better. She even smiles now and then which makes me feel better. It really was a long stretch that Joan was so sick. I sure hope we are all done with that part of Joan's program to get better. Our Grandson James called us tonight to see how Joan was doing and to thank us for sending a project he needed at school. He needed a report on plant life from another state, so we sent him a report on some of Florida's plant life. Our Grandchildren also thought Joan was not feeling well. The young ones know Joan is sick but do not know just how sick she was. We love our whole family. All four of our children and all thirteen of their children [our grandchildren]. We just wish we could be with them more especially when we do not feel well. Oh well, I'm sure we will be on the go again as soon as Joan is feeling all better. I think it is time for me to say goodnight. The eyes are starting to close on me. Will be with you tomorrow. Goodnight.

PS, We are on "vacation" again - Saturday and Sunday. Boy, did last week go fast.

October 18, 2003

Got up about 8:30 AM. Lewis the gardener was coming and I wanted to tell him what to do. Joan was sleeping in, seeing that we did not have any appointments to go to. It is really great that Joan is feeling better, just maybe we can get back to a normal life again. I know she is going to be very tired from the radiation treatment and that she will have a lot more to do when all the treatments are done, but it sure feels good to see the improvement in the way she feels now. When Joan awoke we had breakfast and got ready for our first vacation day to start. Lewis came and I went outside with him for a while. Joan sewed a button on my shirt and did a load of wash, what a slave driver I am. We didn't do to much more except read the newspaper and wait for lunch time. I made tuna salad for lunch with potato chips and some grapes. After lunch I went to the store and also stopped in at our daughter Kim's house to see how the addition to their house was coming along. Joan stayed home and took it easy. Today seemed to be a pretty normal day for us, almost like nothing was wrong at all. I sure hope we have many more days like today. Joan was good. The weather was good. And, even I was good. When I got home I took it easy until it was dinner time. I thought I would make spaghetti and sausage for dinner, which I did and it was pretty good. After dinner we took it easy. We talked and watched T/V for a little while. Joan decided to go to bed and watch the T/V. I went outside and talked to a neighbor for a while. When I came in I thought I would also get comfortable and watch the World Series game. We both got tired and decided to go to sleep. Today was really the best day we had in a very long time. Joan felt good all day and we did some normal things. All in All it was a very good day so I think I will just say goodnight. Goodnight.

October 19, 2003

This is our second day of our "vacation". Hopefully it will be as good as our first day of our two day vacation. We got up at 9:30 AM. We are all slept out, I think. Joan seems to feel the same as yesterday which was very good. I also feel very good, just maybe we can repeat yesterday's performance. Today I need to clean up the garage and Joan is getting the house pretty for our visit from Rose and Joe Nassara. They are going on a cruise that leaves from Fort Lauderdale, FL on Monday. They left Hilton Head SC at 9:00 this morning and will be going right past our exit on I-95 about 4:30 PM, so they are going to stop in for a very short visit to see Joan. Rose just wants to see how Joan is for herself. Rose calls Joan about every week or so, to see how she is doing. Sometimes she will call twice in a week if she thinks Joan was doing badly. I can't imagine not having Rose and Joe as our dearest friends. Really, they are more like family than friends and that's the truth. Rose and Joe also pray a lot for Joan, which means everything to us and brings us even closer to God. Our friendship with Rose and Joe is entwined with our belief in God. This makes it a very special relationship. After Joan talks to Rose she is like a different person and when Joan and I visit with Rose and Joe or just in their company, we both feel the same way. They are very special to us. Joan has no nausea and feels the same as she did yesterday, I do think without pushing it, that we are really on the mend. We will pray that it will stay this way. Rose and Joe, Betty and Frank all arrived at 5:00 PM. Betty and Frank are going on the cruise with Rose and Joe. Betty is Rose's sister and Frank is Betty's husband. Now that the introductions are over, I can tell you that we enjoy Betty and Frank's company also. They are real nice and a pleasure to be with. They all stayed until about 6:30 PM. We had some snacks for them and had a good time just being together. I'm sure Rose and Joe were glad to see that Joan looked as good as she does. The last few days have been good for Joan and I am sure it made her look much better than she had been looking. After they all left Joan and I went out for dinner, we went to the Bob Evans Restaurant for pot roast. It's one of there specialties - very good. After dinner we came right home and settled in for the night; Joan with her shows that she likes while I watched the World Series, game number two. I must say that the last two days have been just great. We felt more like our selves than we have felt in months. I hope and pray that this will continue from now on. I think I will close for tonight and hope for another good day tomorrow and the day after that and on and on, etc, etc. Goodnight.

Radiation: Day Eleven (Third Week)

October 20, 2003

Today is the first day of the third week of Joan's radiation program. We started by getting up at 7:30 AM. We got ourselves ready to go to the Doctor's. We left at 11:00 AM and as usual got to the Doctor's office at 11:45 AM. Joan had the treatment, talked to the Doctor and was ready to go home by 12:45 PM. The Doctor said everything was going according to schedule and he was glad that Joan was handling the radiation treatment without any problems to this point. Tomorrow we need to be at the Doctor's office at 2:00 PM instead of 12:00 PM. They need to make some adjustments with the machine on Joan's body which is normal at this point. We get to sleep a little longer in the morning . Sounds good to me. When we got home from the Doctor's office we had lunch and just sat and talked about things - nothing in particular - just about how we were doing. Joan felt tired and took a nap. I did some paper work and got on the computer for awhile. I think the afternoon went by very quickly, because all of a sudden it was time for dinner. [Time sure does fly by.] Tonight we did what we usually do - watch T/V and go to bed. There was no baseball tonight so I watched whatever Joan was watching. Our daughter Diane called and talked with Joan for almost an hour, I think Diane just wanted to be brought up to date on everything. All our kids call on a regular basis, so we hear from at least one of them daily. This is what keeps us going. Without our Kids and our friends we would be in a real state of depression. It is now late and we are tired so I think we will turn in for the night. Talk with you again tomorrow. OK? Goodnight.

Radiation: Day Twelve

October 21, 2003

Today we do not have to go to the Doctor's office until 2:00 PM. Joan needs to have the adjustments made on the radiation machine and this was when the doctor was able to do it. The morning was as usual get up, shower, get dressed and have breakfast. This gave us time to get some things done before we have to leave. I had to take the Benz. to be looked at so that took most of the time up, when I got home Joan had done some things around the house and was ready to go to the Doctor's. We had lunch first and then left about 1:15 PM to go to the Doctor's. We arrived at the Doctor's about 2:00 PM. There is more traffic at this time than there is when we go in the morning. They took Joan right away and were about to start to re-mark Joan but the Doctor was called to the hospital on an emergency so instead of re-marking Joan they just gave her the regular radiation treatment and said that they would have to re-mark Joan at another time. They will let us know by tomorrow, I'm sure. With the confusion it took a little longer before we were ready to go home. It must have been 3:30 by the time we left the Doctor's office. We arrived home about 4:00 PM. Again the traffic was a lot heavier than we experienced during the morning treatments. After getting home Joan was very tired and needed to take a rest. I needed to go to the store for some food. We were running out of everything. It took me over an hour to shop, mostly because I was also tired and was not moving to fast. When I got home from shopping I took it easy for about an hour and then I started to make dinner. Neither of us were very hungry so I scrubbed the kind of dinner we were going to have and we settled for a sandwich. It was the right decision. Anything more would have been too much. After dinner, which was kind of late, we talked to our kids on the phone and discussed what had happened at the Doctor's. It was now T/V time; Joan with her programs and me with the World Series. Joan fell asleep watching a show and never knew what the ending was. I, on the other hand, watched the whole World Series game right to the end. Now it is time to go to sleep so I will say goodnight. Goodnight.

PS - It is nice seeing Joan do things around the house. It gives me the feeling that she is really getting better. A week ago she did not want to do anything.

Radiation: Day Thirteen

October 22, 2003

Back to our regular schedule; up at 7:30 raring to start the day. Took a shower, got dressed, had breakfast and hung around waiting to leave at 11:00 AM, our normal time. We arrived at the Doctor's office about 11:35 AM, better time than yesterday when we went in the afternoon. Joan again felt good, YEAH. They took Joan right away. They did the radiation treatment and told Joan that they would most likely re-mark her next week. Joan was finished and ready to go at 12:00 PM. I was having a cup of coffee, so Joan had to wait for me. They have the best coffee in the waiting room and every now and then people bring in buns or cookies to go with the coffee. All the patients seem to look out for one another. It's like a bond they all have seeing that they are all having the same or similar problems. They really feel for each other and it shows. On our way home we decided to go to the Caddy dealership and look at a car that just came out - a 2004 model. They call it the S.R.X.. It's a seven passenger and is just beautiful and I mean beautiful. I think we are going to buy it. We will know better when we go back to the dealer tomorrow. We were quite excited about it and I think it was the happiest we have been in a long time. We both had smiles on our faces a mile wide, or so it seemed. After we left the dealer we went right home and had dinner. The dinner I was going to have last night I made tonight; roast chicken, corn and a salad. After dinner we just discussed what we did for the day and we realized that it was a pretty normal day after Joan had her treatment. We both felt pretty good health wise, how about that. I think it is time we turn on the T/V. Joan, to her programs and me to the World Series - game FOUR. Well we will see you tomorrow OK. Goodnight .

Radiation: Day Fourteen

October 23, 2003

We again got up at 7:30 AM, did our normal morning things, had breakfast and just waited around till it was time to go to the Doctor's, which was 11:00 AM. We arrived at the Doctor's at 11:45 AM and they took Joan right away as they always do. Joan felt good and the nurses even mentioned that she looked better than she has been looking. We left the Doctor's office as soon as Joan was finished with her treatment. This was about 12:15 PM. We knew we were going to go to the Caddy dealership to decide what we were going to do about the new car. Well we decided. We bought it and believe it or not, we even took it home with us. It took a long time to do all the paper work and to change the registration, but we got it done and it is now in our garage and it is ours. It has been a long time since we have been this excited, and I think it is just what we needed. For the last two days we thought of nothing else but the car. The change of pace was a great feeling. When we got home it was late and we had not had anything to eat since breakfast. I know I had a headache and I am sure Joan had one too. After we ate we thought it would be a good idea to just relax. We put on the T/V and watched a couple of funny half hour shows. We talked for a while and then decided to go to bed. We are both very tired and need to go to sleep. Will talk to you tomorrow. Goodnight.

Radiation: Day Fifteen

October 24, 2003

Today was the half way mark. That's right, we are half way through our radiation program. Its hard to believe that we only have three more weeks to go. The most wonderful feeling is that Joan has handled the radiation program to this point very well. All the prayers that everyone has said for Joan and I have really made the difference. Of that we are sure. It is just a beautiful feeling to know that so many people and loved ones care that much for Joan's recovery. I'm sure that with all this love everything is going to turn out just right. We got up this morning at the usual time and also arrived at the Doctor's office at the usual time. When we left the Doctor's office [everything went well] we had to go back to the Caddy dealership to finish up some loose ends from buying the car yesterday. The car is now completely ours. When we got home we were very tired and needed a good rest. Last night neither Joan nor I slept to well. I think we were thinking about all we did in buying the car. Joan laid down in the bed and fell sound asleep. I sat in the lounge chair and also fell asleep. Would you believe we slept for two and a half hours. It is now time for dinner and neither of us are very hungry. I think we will just pick on what ever we feel like having and call that dinner for tonight. I guess it is that time T/V and to get ready for bed, so I will sign off for the night. Will talk to you tomorrow. Goodnight.

PS – THANK YOU FOR ALL YOUR PRAYERS. WE COULD NOT HAVE GOTTEN THIS FAR WITHOUT THEM.

How We Feel at This Point

We are now half way through our radiation program and Joan is doing just great. She does not have the nauseous feeling any more and she seems to be handling the radiation very well. Yes, she gets very tired and sleeps a lot but that is par for the course with radiation. As far as any other side effects go, Joan has a little swelling on the left side at the bottom of her rib cage. The Doctor does not know about it yet, but we will tell him on Monday. The swelling only showed up last Friday night. It seems that there have been no other side effects that Joan has experienced to this point. We have been feeling much better emotionally. We are starting to enjoy doing things. Joan, as I have said, is still very tired and we only do what she can handle. But at least we feel like we are getting back to normal. We know that we have a way to go yet before we know we have beaten the cancer. We are thinking very positive and in our minds feel that we have already done that. We will still pray that we did and hope that all the prayers that are being said for Joan will continue. We have no words to thank all of you for your prayers except to say, THANK YOU AND WE LOVE YOU ALL.

October 25 & 26, 2003

These two days are our "vacation" days from the radiation treatment. No treatments and no Doctor's appointments to go to. Just do what we want and when we want to do it. It is also our fifty first anniversary [Sunday the 26th]. Saturday we got up about 9:30 AM, did our normal things to get ready for the day, had breakfast and just took it easy. We had a lot of reading to do about our new car. There is so much equipment and new kind of things to read about that it seems it will take forever to digest it all. I guess the best way to do it is to sit in the car with the book and just try everything. Joan is very excited about the new car. I don't ever remember her being so excited about a car as she is about this one. Could be that she has been in the doldrums for so long that anything good that happens will give her the high she seems to be on. I also am very excited about the car, it really is not a car and it is not really an S.U.V. As they say at the dealership it is their in between change over vehicle. Its called the S.R.X breakthrough by the Cadillac. All I know is it is just what the doctor ordered to take our minds off what has been going on. Most of the day was spent on the car and showing it off, which of course is also a part of getting something new, and a lot of fun. We ended Saturday in the usual way; dinner, T/V and going to bed.

Sunday was the same getting up, doing our thing and having breakfast. The nice thing about today was that it was our fifty first anniversary which, in itself, is quite exciting for us. This is also great for Joan and I because it is another special event that brings us back to being normal again. Life has its downers, but if you try real hard you can overcome them and get back to the way things are really supposed to be - HAPPY. The downers can also be a good learning experience that will just enforce what you really believe in. We also had another real nice thing happen to us today. Joan and I like to go to a restaurant on the ocean in Hutchinson Island, about thirty or so minutes from our home. We were talking to our daughter Doreen in NJ about what we plan to do today and she thought that it would be real nice for us to go there. Both of our daughters Doreen and Diane have been there and liked it just as we do.

Well, when we arrived at the restaurant we were greeted with Hello Mr. and Mrs. Dickson, HAPPY ANNIVERSARY, please come right this way. They brought us to a very nice table overlooking the Ocean just like we would have wanted to do. We wondered how they knew our names and that it was our anniversary. I guess it didn't take us long to figure it out. You got it. Our daughters Doreen and Diane were the culprits. They do many things like this from time to time. Maybe they kinda like their Mom and Dad. Do you think? [Our other children also treat us real special]. We are very fortunate parents.

Well, everyone, we have had a fantastic weekend. With all the good things that have happened to us in the past few days I'm sure we will be on a high for quite a while. We will try to keep it that way. I think I need to call it quits for tonight so I will say goodnight. Goodnight.

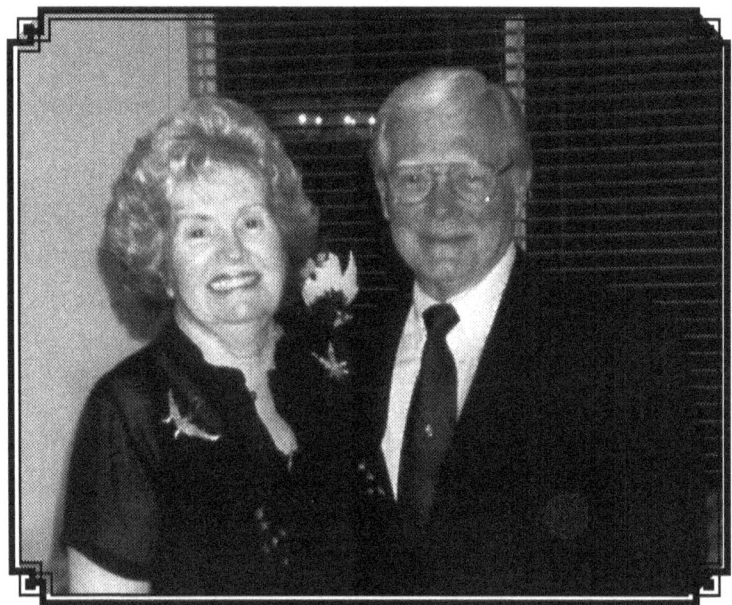

Radiation: Day Sixteen

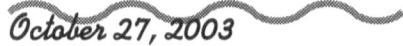

October 27, 2003

Here we go again. This is the start of the second half of our radiation treatments for Joan. We did the first half in, I would say, pretty good shape. The time just seemed to fly by. Today we got up at 7:30 AM, took a shower, got dressed and had our breakfast. We hung around until it was time to go to the Doctor's office, which was 11:00 AM [sound familiar?]. We arrived at the Doctor's office at 11:45 AM and Joan was taken right away. After

Joan had her radiation treatment she told the Doctor about the swelling she had at the bottom of her rib cage, on her left side. The Doctor agreed it was swollen and that he would need to check to make sure it was not a tumor. OK, let's do that, said Joan. The Doctor did a hands on inspection and came to the conclusion that it was most likely the disarrangement of some tendons from all that was done to Joan in that area from the operation. He also said it did not feel like a tumor but he would keep an eye on it for a while to make sure. I guess there will always be something to worry about as we go on with Joan's treatments, but as I said before, we know everything is going to be OK. We left the Doctor's office at about 12:30 PM and thought we would get our new car registered at the gate house where we live. This is important seeing that we live in a gated community and for security reasons every car has to be registered. After we did that we went right home. Joan was rather tired and I had a few things to do this afternoon. After we had lunch Joan laid down for a rest and I made a trip to my Daughter and Tony's condo at the PGA Village. I had to check on some work that was done in their condo. Everything was OK, so I left for home. I have to back track here a little. When Joan and I were on our way home from the Doctor's we did make a stop at a auto supply store to get some mats for the car. The car has mats but Joan likes to have the clear mats to put on the mats that are already there to protect the rugs that came with the car. Next Joan will want every one to take off their shoes so the clear mats will not get dirty. Oh well, cleanliness is next to godliness, so they say. Back to where I was, on my way home from the condo. I stopped at the drugstore to get Joan's prescriptions that the Doctor had ordered for her. When I finally got home it was time to have dinner but again we were not very hungry, so we decided that we would eat later. I guess it was time to take it easy and just watch a show or two on the T/V. While we were watching T/V I made us a snack for dinner; soup and sandwich. We had a pretty full day so I think we will just go to bed and get some sleep. Goodnight.

Radiation: Day Seventeen

October 28, 2003

We had a good nights sleep, I don't think either of us got up more than ounce. It is 7: 00 AM and I am fully awake and ready to start the day. I will wake Joan up about 8: AM and we will start our day, shower, get dressed and have breakfast. After breakfast I needed to go to the bank and handle a couple of things. When I got home Joan was almost ready to go to the Doctor's. Joan looked very nice today, she usually looks nice every day, but for some reason she looks special today. It must be the good night's sleep we had. She feels good too. We left our usual time for the Doctor's office, 11:00 AM, and got there as usual by 11:45 AM. After Joan had her treatment we went up to the second floor in the same building to visit the library that is run by Martin Memorial cancer center. It is comfortable and you can find out most anything you want to know about any kind of cancer there is. I talked to the social worker in charge who is very helpful if you need a question answered. We went to the library to find out what it was all about. We found out that you never need to feel alone when you have an organization like this at your side. All you need to do is say "help" and they are right there to do whatever they can for you. Again, I'll say there are really very good people in this world of ours. I was very impressed with our visit. After our visit we left for home. First we stopped for lunch at the Jenson Ale House - a good place to go for lunch. After lunch we went to our regular Doctor to get our flu shots. We usually get the flu shot before now but the Doctors wanted Joan to wait for a while after her chemo treatments. We are now on our way home with no more stops to make. Even though we had a good nights sleep we are now tired, especially Joan. I think her eyes are at half mast. It is now late afternoon and about the time to think about dinner. I think we will just pick tonight. Our lunch was more than enough so we are not at all Hungary. I think we will say goodnight for today, we will be going to bed early I'm sure. Talk to you tomorrow. Goodnight.

Radiation: Day Eighteen

October 29, 2003

Today I started the day at 6:30 AM. I woke up and have no idea why, it's not only the hour it's I am completely wide awake. Oh well, an early start will not hurt. I have a lot on the agenda for today. I will wake Joan about 8:00 AM to start her day. After I wake Joan, we will get ready for the day, shower, dress and have breakfast. Yes, we left for the Doctor's office on time and arrived on time. Joan had her radiation treatment and we left for home. Joan felt pretty good so we decided to stop at the Treasure Coast

Mall for lunch. We go to the food court, to a diner that has the best Philly Steak sandwiches that you can get. They are really good. We top it off with a soft ice cream cone that is also really good. What's nice about eating at the food court is that you get to watch all the people coming and going and it is like watching a fashion show. You get to see all the different styles that are out there. It really is fun. Nutty, but fun - people are really great. While we were at the mall we went to the AT&T store to get our new cell phone working and also had it registered. It was easier than doing it myself. We left the mall and Joan told me she had an appointment to have her nails done. So, off we went to the nail salon. I'm really very happy that she wants to do these things. To me it means she is really getting better and she is doing what makes her happy. When we got home Joan laid down for a needed rest. I had some paper work to do, so into my office I went. When Joan woke up from her rest we had dinner and just sat around talking until it was time for me to go to the association meeting which started at 7:00 PM. It usually does not last to late. I got home about nine PM and hung out with my wife. I bet you can't guess what we did. Yep, you got that right, watched T/V and then to bed. We have to go to the Doctor's early tomorrow. We need to go to both Doctor's, first for a blood test and then to the radiation treatment. So we will say goodnight for now. Goodnight.

PS – Today was a very good day, it felt like we were kids again - just on a date and really enjoying ourselves. Maybe we can make every day like this one - at least we can give it a try.

Radiation: Day Nineteen

October 30, 2003

Today we need to leave a little early so we can go to Doctor Iannotti for a blood test. This needs to be done before we go to Joan's radiation treatment at 12:00 PM. Doctor Griffis wants Joan's blood levels to be in good shape so he can continue with the radiation. We could not be happier with the way all of Joan's Doctor's are handling her programs. It is a real team effort by, what we feel, is the best and most professional Doctors in each of their fields. We could not be in better hands and we thank all of them from the bottom of our hearts. This also goes for all those that work along side them. If you have confidence in your doctors and all those that they work with, half of the battle is won. If you honestly do what they tell you to do, the other half will also be won. After we left the Doctor's we went home to take a rest, and then get ready to go to dinner with four of our dear friends and neighbors. Two of them are moving so we thought it would be great to spend some time with them for dinner. They are only moving about three hours away so we are sure we will be seeing them again. After dinner we all went home. We had a great time and a lot of laughs. Joanne and Fred both were tired so it was better that we called it a day. Fred is facing an operation very soon and he needs to take it easy. Joanne also needs her rest. Joan and I watched a little T/V and turned in for the night. I guess we will say goodnight. Goodnight.

PS – Another good day. Joan did good.

Radiation: Day Twenty

October 31, 2003 - Happy Halloween!

I had to get up early today. I needed to take the new car to the dealers for a minor problem. They said they would have it ready after 3:00 PM today. They gave me a loaner so I could take Joan to the Doctor's. When I returned home from the dealers it was only 9:30 AM, which gave us plenty of time to get to Joan's appointment for her radiation. We had breakfast and than left for the Doctor's. When we walked into the waiting room it really looked like Halloween. It was all decorated and they also had hot cider, coffee, cake, and a ton of cookies. They also had another ton of all kinds of candy. Like I said they really have a genuine feeling for all of their patients, They make you feel like you are coming to visit friends, not just going to the Doctor's. After we left the Doctor's office we headed home. It only took about one half hour, which was about the best time ever. Once home we had lunch and talked about putting up some decorations for Halloween. The outside of our home had already been decorated for a couple of days. Our daughter and the grandchildren are coming over tonight like they do every Halloween, so we get a chance to see the kids all dressed up in their costumes, which is always great. Joan is doing pretty good. The only thing that bothers her is she feels a bit achy and a little feeling of nausea now and then. And, of course, she is always very tired. We know that being tired is from the radiation, the nausea and being achy we couldn't figure out until we remembered that we just had our flu shots and this could be a reaction from the shot. We will ask the Doctor. Joan took a rest in the afternoon and I went back to the dealers to get our new car. On my way home I stopped at the hair salon where Joan and I get our hair done. Joan once a week and me about every two months. Getting her hair done every week is something that Joan has been doing since we have been in Florida. I must say, Joan's hair always looks just great and Joan feels real good about it. When I walked in to the salon they gave me a great big greeting and they all wanted to know how Joan was. I call them now and then to keep them posted on Joan's condition, but I guess it was nicer that they saw one of us. When I got home Joan was asleep so I took it easy for a little while. All of a sudden it was time for dinner, so I had to get cooking. Joan was now awake and came into the kitchen to help me. After we had dinner we watched T/V and just waited for Kim and the kids to arrive. Kim, John and the four grand kids arrived about 8:30 PM. We had a great time seeing all the costumes. We had cider, doughnuts and some large Halloween cookies which were real good. Our next door neighbors brought over some candy for the children like they do every year. Of course the kids all like that. It was now about 9:30 PM and Kim John and the kids still had to visit Johns parents so they could see the kids all dressed up. Everyone left so Joan and I got ready for bed and watch a little T/V. Tonight it was a constant show of the original cast of the Munsters. It was fun to watch for a while but we did switch to the programs we usually watch and then went to sleep. It was another good day for both Joan and I. Things are really getting better and seem to be getting back to being more normal, at least we are starting to have fun back in our lives. I guess it is time to say goodnight. Goodnight.

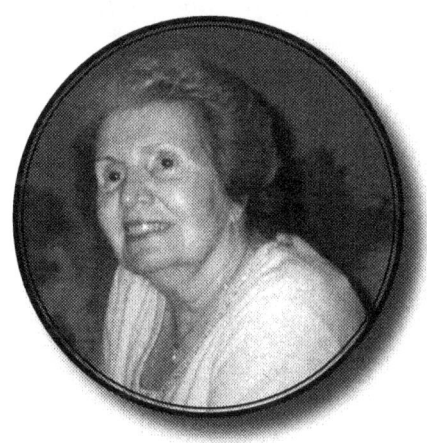

Voice of the Children

How did you talk to your children about this situation?
My children Kristie (25) Kerri (22) and A.J. (18) are much older then the rest of my parents' grandchildren so they understood exactly what was going on. They felt like my husband and myself, that it was very difficult not being there to help them through this. I don't think that any of them felt she would not get through it. They never talked to me about her dying. They always were talking about her getting better. My daughter Kerri probably understood what her grandmother was going through the most, as she was best friends with my best friend's daughter who died from breast cancer. *Diane*

My children range from the ages of 2 to 14 years old, so we got a wide range of questions. My two year old was only one when this happened so of course she didn't know what was going on. My seven year old was very curious but more so about why Grandma was loosing her hair and why she wasn't feeling good for so long. My two older children understood and were very concerned as to when Grandma would feel better. *Kim*

We made sure that our kids understood what was happening to their grandmother in Florida and that they should make sure they prayed for her to get better. We didn't have to explain much to them because at the same time my mom was going through this in Florida, My mother-in-law (who lives with us in PA) was going through a very similar procedure. Within days of my mother's surgery, my mother-in-law had a cancerous lump removed from her neck and chest. Our kids experienced what my mother was going through, in person, with their other Grandmother who also had to go through the radiation and chemotherapy treatments at the same time. *Ken*

My children are at an age where they are somewhat understanding of what goes on cancer. It's probably discussed more then we would like to think. My eleven year old was especially concerned and prayed everyday for grandma to get better. *Doreen*

November

November 1, 2003

It is hard to believe that we are already into November. Time seems to go by so fast, in one way while Joan is still in treatment it probably is OK, but as soon as Joan is all better it better slow down. We need to do a lot of catching up and want all the time we can get to do it.. being that it is Saturday we did not have to get up early. It sure felt good to sleep in for awhile. This is what we call our two day "vacation". No Doctor's or appointments to go to. We got up at 9:00 AM, Lewis the gardener and Richard the man that does just about anything will be here at 10:30 AM so we need to be finished with getting ready for the day and have our breakfast . Joan seems to feel OK today. She still feels a little achy and a bit nauseous from what we think is due to the flu shots, if it does not pass in a couple of days we will really have to find out where it is coming from. The swelling that Joan has under her rib cage seems to be getting better. It is not as swollen as it was which is a good sign. It seems that the worst is behind us, at least we hope so. I feel my beautiful lady is just doing fine. I am really very proud of her. She has really kept her spirits up and tried hard to over come all the things she has had to endure. Thinking positive is a real must if you want to get through all the procedures that it takes to get well from this illness. The rest of Saturday for Joan was just taking it easy. She wrote some cards and watched the T/V in between a couple of naps. I did some work outside in my garden, and sort of cleaned up around the outside of the house. About 5:00 PM after I cleaned up from being outside, I did not feel to good for some reason. My right inside ear was hurting along with a problem swallowing; sort of a sore throat but not real bad. Just enough to be uncomfortable. My body did not feel like doing anything but lying down. I took a couple of aspirin and just took it easy for awhile. It seemed I could not get enough energy to even make dinner, so we just had some good old chicken soup - the cure-all for everything. Needless to say, the rest of the day was not going to be too exciting, We watched T/V for about an hour, or I should say Joan watched T/V - I sort of fell sound asleep in the lounge chair. We decided it was time for me to go to bed and that is just what I did. Talk with you tomorrow OK?

Goodnight.

November 2, 2003

Today I thought I would wake up and be a very sick guy. The way I felt when I went to bed last night indicated I had the flu or even something worse. Much to my surprise I got out of bed and I felt pretty good, I did not have an ear problem or a throat problem or any other kind of problem except for a body that ached like I just ran a marathon race. Last night when I went to bed I had all of the above problems including the achy body. I guess it was still the reaction from the flu shot, or maybe it was that I had a talk with you know who, and I asked him to please keep me well so I can take care of my Joan while she is going through her sickness. I kind of think that is really why I OK today. At least I think so. Heck, I know so. I woke Joan up about nine thirty AM and she was also very surprised that I was even up. We decided that with what happened last night, we would just keep a low profile for today. Again, I know she was relieved that I was OK. Joan does really not like it when I do not feel good. Like I said, we will keep a low profile for the day and do as little as possible. Joan feels pretty good, so maybe we can just enjoy each other for the day. We will talk with you tomorrow.

Goodnight.

Radiation: Day Twenty-one

November 3, 2003

Today we are back on our regular schedule. Our "vacation" days are over until next week. I got up at 7:30 AM and got things going to start the day. I woke Joan up at 8:00 AM so she can start her day. We also needed to be up early today because Carol was coming to clean at 9:00 AM and we needed to tidy up before she got here. [only kidding]. After breakfast we left for the Doctor's office for Joan's radiation treatment. Today is the day the Doctor goes over everything with Joan and lets her know how she is doing. If he has anything really important to say he will invite me in to talk also. Today he told Joan that the swelling under her ribs seem to be much better and not as swollen. This pretty much eliminates the idea of the possibility that there was a tumor present in that area. Very good news, thank you God. The Doctor told Joan that he was adding three more day's to her radiation program to be on the safe side. He said he usually likes to do thirty three days instead of thirty days as we thought it was going to be. Anything he wants to do to make sure that Joan is going to be better is very OK with us. After we left the Doctor's office we went straight home. We got home at 1:00 PM which is just a little later than we usually get home. I guess it was a little longer talking to the Doctor. We had lunch and than Joan thought she would take a rest. Joan feels pretty good and so do I. Things are looking up. I know I keep talking on how good things are going, and it really is and maybe we are on a high and seem to be anticipating the outcome of Joan's illness, but we have a lot of faith and we just feel that things are going to be just fine. We will still pray and hope everyone else will pray with us, not only for Joan but for everyone that has been stricken with this terrible sickness.

After Joan woke up from her nap we watched a little T/V and we also talked about what happened today at the Doctor's. We always talk out what the Doctor tells us so we are sure we understand what he said. If we don't understand anything we jot it down and ask him the next day. This way we are sure of what we are doing and that we do everything he wants us to do. It is getting to be dinner time so I better get moving and make us something to eat. We had dinner and I am sure we will do a little reading and then turn in for the night.

Bet you thought I was going to say watch T/V and go to bed. They say variety is the spice of life. We will watch T/V tomorrow night.

Goodnight.

Radiation: Day Twenty-two

November 4, 2003

There is no rush to go anyplace today. Our appointment for Joan's radiation is not until 3:00 PM this afternoon, so we get to sleep in for a bit. I, on the other hand, had to be at the bank for a 9:00 AM appointment. I was only gone for about one hour. When I returned home Joan was up and ready to start the day. We had breakfast and we both looked over some medical bills that we received and did not look just right. We made some calls and I think we have them all straightened out; at least it looks like it is. The medical bills are another whole part of all that is going on with Joan's illness. I think we need a CPA just to figure out what they are doing. Oh well, # 1 is the state of Joan's health. Everything else can [jolly well] wait. I'm sure it will get settled to everyone's satisfaction. [Insurance companies are confusing.]

After lunch Joan and I left for the Doctor's to get her radiation treatment at 3:00 PM. We got there just in time and they were all ready to start. Joan's appointment was at 3:00 PM because Joan had to have some adjustments made by the Doctor and this was the time he could do it.

First they gave Joan the radiation treatment; then they made the adjustments. The whole procedure took about thirty five minutes. [more drawings and road maps] We left for home about 3:45 PM and went right home. Joan was very tired and did not want to do anything else. When we got home Joan took a nap and did not wake up until dinner time. I was a little tired myself so I ordered dinner from the Italian restaurant - pasta and salad - pretty good but we were not too hungry. [It was an effort just to eat]. I think tonight will be another early go to bed night. So I think I will say good night now. Goodnight. PS – yes we did watch a little T/V and than went to sleep early.

Radiation: Day Twenty-three

November 5, 2003

Going back to last night, I woke up about 3:00 AM, what seemed to be for no reason. I was very restless and I had a hard time getting relaxed enough to get back to sleep. At 4:00 AM, I woke up again feeling the same way as before. After tossing for awhile I thought I better check on Joan.

Sure enough, she was awake and just sitting in the bath room. I guess I should have checked on her at three because she had been awake since then. At three I did not hear anything or see any lights on, so I had no idea that Joan was not asleep. When I asked Joan what was wrong, she told me that she was very nauseous and she could not sleep because she felt like she was going to throw up. Joan did not throw up but we stayed awake until almost 5:30 waiting to see if she was going to become ill. We finally dozed off and by that time it was almost time to get up for the day. We have no idea what caused Joan to feel the way she did. It was the same feeling that she would get when she was on the chemo program, I guess it will be another question for the Doctor when we see him today. We are now up for the day, or I should say I'm up and Joan is still asleep. I had to go back to the dealer at 8:30 AM this morning so they could put the part they ordered in the car. When I came home at 9:30, Joan was awake and just waiting for me to get back. We had breakfast and got ready to leave for the Doctor's for Joan's radiation treatment. We arrived on time and Joan had her treatment right on time. Joan asked the nurse about how she felt last night and the nurse said that the chemo was not completely out of her system and she could still get a feeling of nausea. I guess we were second guessing the program again. The nurse said she would tell the Doctor so he could tell us tomorrow. [The Doctor was not available today] The nurse said not to worry as long as you feel OK now and Joan does feel OK now. [So we won't worry.] Joan has been doing so good that we felt that part of the program was behind us. [Wrong.] I guess you just have to go with the flow and whatever happens, will happen. We will handle it just like we have everything else, we will not let anything change our minds about Joan getting all better. When we left the Doctor's we went right home. Joan was really Very tired and so was I. I guess you can't stay up half the night and not be tired at some point the next day. We had some lunch and talked about what the nurse had said until Joan's eyes started to look like tiny slits. Joan went to bed for a much needed nap and I even felt like a nap but had to go to a meeting at the club house for the Isle of Granada which was at 3:30 PM. The meeting lasted until 5:00 PM. When I got home Joan was still napping so I decided to start dinner and wake Joan when it was all ready. I made my favorite meal - Pork Chop Stew. It is a meal I made up and everyone seems to like. I woke Joan up and to my disappointment found out that she did not feel well again. She felt the same as last night

- nauseous and all. Of course she was not in any way interested in the stew. I made Joan some soup which she just about handled eating. After dinner, such as it was, all Joan wanted to do was to go back to bed, which she did. I did manage to eat some stew but I sort of lost my appetite to. Oh well, there is always tomorrow. I am sure that Joan will be feeling better and maybe we can get back to normal again. There wasn't much more that happened today so I might as well say goodnight. Goodnight.

I'm sure we will be doing better by tomorrow.

Radiation: Day Twenty-four

November 6, 2003

This morning we got up at 7:30 AM. I Should have said I got up, Joan slept until 8:30 AM. When she woke up she was better than last night but still had the nausea feeling; not as bad but it was still there. After we got ourselves ready for the day and had our breakfast it was just about time to leave for the Doctor's. We left for the Doctor's at 11:00 AM and arrived at his office at 11:45 AM as we usually do. They took Joan right away but for some reason it took a little longer than usual. Joan told the nurse that she felt a little better but not much. The nurse did tell the Doctor and he confirmed what the nurse said yesterday. Until all the treatments are over Joan could still get any of the side effects like nausea, getting tired, achy and just not feeling well. It was real nice for the couple of weeks that Joan seemed to have no side effects except being real tired. I am sure it will be that way soon again. After we left the Doctor's we went right home. We had lunch and Joan thought she had better lie down for a nap or she would fall asleep at the table. Sleeping at the table I have done - it's not too comfortable. While Joan was napping I went to the dealer to pick up our new car that was being serviced. We were anxious to get it back seeing that they had it for two days. Joan and I really love our new car, it is probably the most excited we have ever gotten about a car.

It also came at a time when we have not had to much excitement in our lives. After looking over the car we just hung out together doing much of nothing. We're good at that and have had a lot of experience doing it lately. Joan is still not feeling to good so she went back to lie down and probably will fall asleep. I needed to go to the food store for a couple of things we needed. It also gave me a chance to get Joan some of her favorite ice cream for a treat later tonight. I hope she can eat it but if she can't it will keep for another day. I don't care how sick you might feel, ice cream always makes you feel better. We kind of went light for dinner seeing that Joan's stomach is not too good. I was supposed to go to a Granada meeting tonight but I cancelled it to stay with Joan. I do not like leaving her when she might throw up, she sort of gets faint when she throws up. [I'm sorry I'm talking about this but it is what's happening] and I'm afraid she might fall over.. I think tonight is about finished for the two of us so I will say goodnight. Goodnight.

Radiation: Day Twenty-five

November 7, 2003

Today ends week five of the radiation program, we have one more week and about three or more days left and that should be it for the radiation program. We of course will be talking with the Doctors as to what happens next. I'm sure they will have something in mind as to what Joan has to do and when she needs to do it. I know whatever they have in mind, I will be right with Joan all the way. As you might have figured out, what happens to Joan is also happening to me. Today was the same as almost every other day, we did our thing in the morning and left for the Doctor's office for Joan's radiation treatment.. When we got to the Doctors we had to wait for Joan to be taken, it seems that the radiation machine broke down and they had to double up on the other machine with all the patients. This was a first but it was not a bad wait. I think it took about twenty minutes extra and we were on our way back home. They are very efficient and are able to handle any emergency that comes along. If the whole world worked as well as this cancer center, we [the world] would be in great shape. When we arrived home we had lunch and just decided to sit for awhile. Joan was still not feeling to good so she went to lie down and take a rest. Along with the nausea Joan is also experiencing some redness on her body where they are treating her with the radiation. The nurses could not believe that the redness did not start before this. I guess Joan lucked out as far as that went. The redness is sort of irritating and a bit uncomfortable. The nurses told Joan to use some aloe cream on the areas that are bothering her. The Doctor recommended the use of 1% Hydrocortisone on the skin for relief by applying the cream four times a day. He cautioned not to apply just before the radiation treatment. While Joan was resting I went to Home Depot for some light bulbs for the garage. I was back home in about 45 minutes and Joan was just starting to move around. I asked Joan what she would like for dinner and I think she said nothing. Well, I made her some soup and much to her surprise she finished it all. Joan has been eating well until she started with the nauseous feeling again. I can't say that I blame her when the stomach is not feeling well, you really do not want to put anything in it. I think I remember saying that before. In fact I know I did. After dinner all Joan wanted to do was to lie down again. She is really tired and a little uncomfortable from the redness on her body where they do the radiation. If I could I would take the pain for her, but seeing that that is impossible to do, I will just try to make her as comfortable as I can. I think Joan has really had it for the night and I am also kind of falling apart. Guess we will say goodnight. Goodnight.

PS - Tomorrow we will be on a two day vacation again.

November 8, 2003

Vacation day # 1 - We slept in this morning. I think it was about 9:30 AM when we woke up. Joan had a pedicure at 11:15 AM and like her nail appointments she does not want to miss doing the toes. Believe it or not I kind of like going with Joan to the nail salon. They are a real great bunch of gals and they treat me almost like I'm one of them. I don't remember going anyplace and laughing as much as I do when I go there. Its like going to a men's barber shop only funnier. We did our thing and had breakfast before going to the salon. When we came home Joan and I thought we would spend most of the day just learning every thing we could about our new car. It has so much equipment that we will be lucky to learn half of the things it has. I'm sure that's pushing it a bit. I don't think we will get more than three or four things under our belts for the day. It really doesn't matter, we just will like learning it together. We might have to go to our neutral corners now and then but we will have fun. We did eat today; breakfast was at our regular time and lunch and dinner were kind of put together. We didn't starve that's for sure. Tonight we will most likely watch T/V and turn in early, but before we do I need to call the kids in PA and NJ to let them know how there Mom is doing. They all call one day and I call them the next day. We all pretty much know what's going on every day. I guess we will turn in for tonight. It's been a good day. Goodnight.

PS - Joan felt a little better today than she has been feeling. Still nauseous but not as bad.

November 9, 2003

Vacation day # 2. We thought we would sleep in for a while, but for some reason we got up at 8:30 AM and could not get back to sleep. We had a good breakfast and just sat around reading the Sunday newspaper. We than decided we would pick up where we left off yesterday, learning about the things in our new car. Today we put things that we had in our old cars into the new car. After that we started on the audio part of the car which is going to take a bit of reading to figure it out. Maybe it would be a good idea if we watched golf for a while and read about the audio system later. Good Idea. After we watched golf it was about time for dinner. We for some reason were both on the tired side. I really do not think we are going to be up to doing to much tonight. It has been rather a lazy day for both of us. We probably will turn in early tonight and get a good nights sleep. Joan still feels a bit nauseous and very, very tired. Other than that she seems to be OK. Tomorrow we will be starting what was to be our last week of radiation. It seems that the time is just flying by. After the finish of this week Joan still will have to do three more days of radiation that the Doctor added to her program. I'm sure the next week and a half will also fly by. I am still holding up, but will be glad when all the running will be finished. No matter how much we have to do and how tired we might get, it is all very much worth going through if my Joan is OK. I think it would be very good if I just say we'll see you tomorrow and say goodnight. Goodnight.

Radiation: Day Twenty-six

November 10, 2003

Up at 8:30 AM, showered, got dressed and had our breakfast. We are now ready to leave for the Doctor's office as soon as it is 11:00 AM. We arrived at the Doctor's our regular time 11:45 AM and they were all ready for Joan. After Joan's radiation treatment she had a talk with Doctor Griffis. Joan asked the Doctor what will be on the agenda after the radiation treatments are all done, The Doctor said we will talk about that when we finish the last treatment. He did say that Joan will have to go back to Doctor Iannotti, the chemo Doctor, after radiation is done. I'm sure we will have a talk with all three Doctor's as to what is going to be next. We will wait and see. We also will be praying that there will be no more chemo. Joan is very tired again today, actually more so the last two days than she has been right along. Joan has also been a little more depressed than she has been for a while. I think it is because we are drawing to a close with the treatments and she does not know what is next. I believe that the Doctor's will tell us that there will be a few tests that Joan will need to see how things are. I am also sure that after the tests, we will be told every thing is A-OK and that all Joan will have to do is to come in for follow up checks on a regular basis. Joan will be OK - I'm sure. She has been very strong through everything so far and after we talk a bit she will be just as strong as she has always been. We are very attached and plan on doing a lot of things for a long time to come. When we got home from the Doctor's we had some lunch, and Joan took a nap. While Joan was napping I went to Home Depot to pick up a few things. After I got home I sort of just took it easy for a while. I will let Joan sleep for a little while longer at least until we are ready to have dinner. After dinner we watched the Wheel of Fortune show, which was being shown in New York City.

It was a repeat of parts of old shows and was very funny. It sort of got some laughs from Joan which was good to see. The rest of the night was more T/V and early to bed again. I'll be back tomorrow. Goodnight .

Radiation: Day Twenty-seven

November 11, 2003

After getting up and getting ready for the day, we left for the Doctor's office to have Joan's radiation treatment. It was a very quick treatment, they only did the area they marked the other day which was right over the incision of the operation to remove the tumor. There were no pictures taken, so Joan was out and ready to go before I got a chance to finish my coffee. We went right home, had lunch and just took it easy for the rest of the afternoon. Joan feels pretty good today; only has a small amount of nausea. Maybe the nausea is going to stop. We sure hope so. Joan is really growing a new head of hair, it is really starting to come in and, believe it or not, it is black and white, not gray but white. I would say that in a couple of weeks she will need to go to Neil to have something done with it. You can tell Joan is very pleased that she is getting her hair back. It really does not matter what color as long as it is hair. When Joan's hair is all in I'm sure that Neil will make it look just like Joan wants it to look. We really have been taking it easy today, and now it is time to have dinner. Dinner tonight will be pasta, which we have at least one time a week. I like pasta but Joan is not that crazy about it. After dinner Joan went to bed and watched T/V and I wanted to do some reading for a while. I will join Joan a little later and then we will retire for the night see you all tomorrow. Goodnight.

Radiation: Day Twenty-eight

November 12, 2003

Time is really going by very fast. After today there are only two more days scheduled per the original schedule for the radiation treatments. There will be three more radiation days next week that the Doctor had added to Joan's treatment schedule to be on the safe side. It feels like we just started with the radiation and here we are almost at the end of the program. To be very honest, outside of Joan getting super tired as a side effect of the radiation and a small amount of discomfort from redness that the radiation leaves on the body, it has not been all that bad. Six and a half weeks seems to be a long time especially going every day. It took us about three hours driving to having the procedure and driving home again. The total treatment days will have been thirty three. We did not have to go on Saturdays and Sundays. Actually the time it took and the procedure itself was not as bad as we anticipated. I know I said this before but I will say it again; The Doctors and all of their staff almost made this a pleasant experience. The only thing that kept it from being a pleasant experience was the reason that we were there. Everyone including the other patients were so pleasant and outgoing that it truly made the whole episode very easy to do. We both mean that from the bottom of our hearts. We will always pray for all at the Martin Memorial Cancer Center. I thank you all for taking care of my Joan. I know I didn't start this day as usual but we did get up, showered, dressed and had our breakfast. The rest of the day was, going to radiation and coming home from radiation. We also had lunch, dinner, watched T/V, took it easy, talked, and went to bed. Goodnight.

Radiation: Day Twenty-nine

November 13, 2003

This morning I am starting in the right order. We got up about 8:30 AM, a little later than usual. We took a shower, got dressed and had our breakfast. I am now back on track. We left for the Doctor's office at 11:00 AM on the button and arrived at his office at 11:45 AM, also on the button. Joan's radiation treatment was only about ten minutes just like the last couple of days. When we left the Doctor's office we went right home. We had lunch and just hung out until Kim, our daughter, called and said that she was going to stop in about 3:00 PM and visit for a while. She will have Mandy and Sierra with her, which pleased us to no end. When Kim arrived we just sat around, talked and played with our Grandkids. Kim and I decided to see how the T/V in the new car worked. Kim got it working in no time while I watched over her shoulder as to how she did it. I'm real good at that - watching that is. Joan was taking care of the kids while Kim and I were in the garage. Joan did real good with the kids. Kim, Mandy and Sierra could only stay for about an hour. Sammie and Justin were due home and Kim wanted to be there when they got home. After Kim and the kids left, Joan and I took a little rest until it was time for dinner. Joan was feeling pretty good both today and yesterday. She did not have any nausea at all. She has been very tired but as long as she is not nauseous she can handle it OK. After dinner we did our usual, watched T/V and just took it easy until we went to bed. It seems we both get real tired when we watch T/V lately. We just keep falling asleep and never see the end of anything we are watching. It must be time to say goodnight, so I will say Goodnight.

Radiation: Day Thirty

November 14, 2003

We got up about 8:00 AM, got ourselves ready for the day and had breakfast. We had to leave early today. Joan had to go to Doctor Iannotti's office for a blood test which she has to have about every ten days. We had to be there at 11:30 AM, which meant we needed to leave home at 10:45 AM. It took us almost thirty minutes for the blood test. They were very busy. After the blood test we went down stairs to the radiation center for

Joan's radiation treatment. They took Joan right away and had her all finished in about ten minutes. They are really fast. Today was our last scheduled appointment for radiation on Joan's program, but we need to do three more treatments next week. Doctor Griffis wants the extra treatments just to be sure. After the next three treatments we will find out what's next for us to do. It sure will be nice not having to take the trip to Stuart every day. After leaving the Doctor's office we went straight home, had lunch and just sat around discussing what we thought would be our next move. I guess we will just have to find out from the Doctor's what it will be. We think Joan will have a short break and then start with some kind of testing to see just how things are. We will wait and see what they say. The rest of the day for Joan was to take a nap, she is really tired. I had to go to a Granada Landscaping meeting at 3:30 PM. The meeting was all about a new program. that the Isle of Granada signed up for, to enhance everyone's landscaping. We were going to go to Bob Evans for dinner tonight but when I got home Joan did not look like she could make it out our front door, so we had Chinese instead. The Chinese was good and we were glad that we ate in. Tonight, I'm sure will be a very early night for the both of us. We are tired. I almost forgot we are going to be on a two day vacation tomorrow. I think we will sleep most of the morning as no one is scheduled all day tomorrow and Luise is coming Sunday instead of Saturday. I think it is that time, so I will say goodnight. Goodnight.

November 15, 2003

Day # 1 of our two day vacation from shots and Doctors and radiation treatments. We just slept until the eyes decided to open. I believe that was about 10:30 AM. When we got out of bed we got ready for the day, showered, got dressed and had breakfast. After breakfast I decided to re-grout the shower floor tiles. There were about six or eight tiles that were getting cracks in the old grout. If I say so myself I did a pretty nice job. Joan not wanting to help me grout did a few things around the house, such as the wash and just generally pick up and straighten up the house. She feels pretty good today and seemed to have enough energy to do a few things. I 'm sure it will be take a nap time soon, but she is gaining on it, she seems to be getting short bursts of energy from someplace. Today is just the most beautiful day we have had in a long time. It is in the high seventies with a cool breeze blowing. I turned off the A/C and opened all the windows to air out the house. Did it ever feel great. I was going to do some other projects around the house but decided it would be real nice if Joan and I just enjoyed the weather and maybe even sat out on the patio and looked at our gardens. It's been a long time since we have just enjoyed our yard. We had lunch rather late, so I can imagine what time we will have dinner. Late afternoon, when we had had enough of looking at our garden, I decided to answer my grandson Ryan's letter to me for Veteran's Day. He had a lot of questions that I had to answer. I'm sure it was a school project because I must send my letter to his school address not to his address. I think this is a great project and I am sure all the children that are doing it will learn a lot from it. [The project was to send a letter to a veteran of any war.] It is now dinner time and neither Joan nor I are the least bit hungry and might not be for quite a while. Oh well, we can always have a snack later. Joan took a look at my letter to our Grandson and made some corrections in spelling for me. It would have been embarrassing to send it to the school if the spelling was not correct. I have a habit when I write to not think of anything but what I am writing and figure I can correct everything later. Joan was a teacher for a long time and is forever correcting me when it comes to doing something the right way. I know she is right and that she is also very good at picking up mistakes. I know it is the teacher in her and is very hard for her to overlook something that is wrong. Thank God for teachers. Without them, where would we be. We finally got a little hungry so I made us some soup with French bread and butter. It tasted great and was just what we felt like. We eat a lot of soup and I am sure it is good for us. We have not been doing too much exercising so we really do not need to many heavy meals. Today has been a good day. The weather was good and Joan was also good. She felt pretty normal and had some pep. We will, I'm sure, watch some T/V and then go to sleep or maybe go to sleep while watching T/V. Goodnight.

November 16, 2003

Good morning! It is another great day out. The weather is just like yesterday - high seventies and a nice cool breeze. I think we most likely will do the same as we did yesterday. We are in the second day of our vacation and really enjoying it. Nothing to do except enjoy our home. I think sometimes we forget just how nice we really have it. We are always looking for something to do when all we have to do is look around us and enjoy what we have. We made a nice breakfast and read the paper for almost an hour and a half. We can see our yard from the breakfast table which makes for a real relaxing atmosphere. After breakfast Joan did a few things around the house and I went outside to see how Luise was doing. He came today instead of yesterday. Yesterday was his little girl's fourth birthday so they had a party for her and of course he could not miss that. We did not do to much for the rest of the day except just enjoy not having to go anywhere. Dinner time came. We ate and went right back to doing nothing. I guess tonight we will watch some T/V and call it a night. There are only a couple of shows on Sunday night that we like, so I'm sure we will go to bed early. Have a good night. Goodnight.

PS - Joan did great today.

Radiation: Day Thirty-one

November 17, 2003

Today we do not have to go to radiation until 4:00 PM. I had an important meeting to go to for the PGA Castle Pines Association, of which we are members. This has to do with the Condo that we own there. The radiation Doctor understood and rescheduled our appointment for later in the day. As I told you, the Doctors and their staff are very sensitive to what ever we want to do and they will help in any way they can. I'm sure it changed their schedule a bit, but as I said they are very kind people. When I came home from the meeting Joan was still asleep. She was kind of tired when we went to bed last night, which I'm sure is from the radiation, so I let her sleep as long as she wanted. It is now about noon time and time for lunch. Joan is awake and ready to do whatever I want. She must be half asleep yet. After lunch we did a little Christmas shopping, looking in the papers and advertising books sent to us. We did find a few things that we will check out. Maybe after we go to Joan's radiation treatment we will stop at the mall, which is on our way home. When Joan was finished with her radiation treatment we had a talk with the Doctor. He said when we are done with Wednesday's radiation treatment we will be given an appointment to see Doctor Iannotti, the chemo doctor. Doctor Iannotti I'm sure will have something for Joan to do like a test of some kind, as long as it is not more chemo we will be very happy. Doctor Griffis wants Joan back to see him when Doctor Iannotti is done. I'm sure Doctor Vopal will also want to see

Joan at some point. We will take one thing at a time. I believe things are starting to wind down a little, we are very glad and a little nervous at the same time. It has been nine months that Joan has been in treatment to overcome the cancer that she was diagnosed with. It is hard to believe that that much time has gone by and the only thing that I can think of doing is to cry. Why, I don't know. I guess it is because in my heart I know Joan is now going to be OK. No one has said that yet but I know it is true. After leaving the Doctor's office we did stop at the mall and did some Christmas shopping. We came up with some good ideas and feel that we at least got a start on the list we have. We have four children, their four spouses and thirteen grandchildren on the top of our list to do. We are just very happy that we are going to be able to do it. And that's for sure. When we left the mall we stopped for dinner, and just relaxed. I think it was about seven o'clock PM when we got home. I know Joan was very tired and I guess I was too. We have a lot of things to think about, but as they say, there is always tomorrow. I will say goodnight now, OK? Goodnight.

Radiation: Day Thirty-two

November 18, 2003

Today we kind of overslept a little. We normally get up at 7:30 AM but today we got up at 8:30 AM. It was no big deal because we do not have to leave until 11:00 AM. We might have to rush a little, but like I said, no big deal. We left after breakfast for the Doctor's office and arrived right on time at 11:45 AM. Our appointment is at 12:00 PM. The treatment was a quick one, so we were ready to go home by 12:15 PM. On our way home we stopped at our daughter Kim's house for a short visit. We have not been to Kim's house for a while, and were really excited to see how much progress they made with the addition they are putting on the house. They are adding a huge family room to the first floor and a bedroom, bathroom and office to the second floor. It is a large undertaking seeing that they are doing it themselves with the help of John's father and brother. It is only being done on week ends and after work during the week. John is very talented with most everything he does and has no fear of trying just about anything. They plan on having the whole addition done before Christmas. I'm sure, knowing my son-in-law, it will be done before Christmas. When we got home we ate lunch, talked a bit and decided that Joan had better lie down or she will fall asleep standing up. It is hard to believe that tomorrow will be Joan's last radiation treatment. The time really flew by, and as time consuming as it was, it was not all that bad. Joan got very tired through out the whole procedure but that was to be expected. Also Joan only had a minimum of discomfort, which surprised us and the Doctor. The discomfort was from the skin irritation of which Joan had very little. Joan did lie down to take a nap. I did some reading and paper work which is something I guess I will always have to do. I woke Joan up just before dinner. If I hadn't, she would most likely have slept until tomorrow morning. After dinner we watched T/V [what else] until it was time to go to bed. I think I will sleep real good tonight. After all of Joan's treatments are over and if the Doctor's say it is OK, I think we will get into some kind of exercise to put us back in shape. I really think it would be good for us. Well, I think it is time to say goodnight. Goodnight.

Radiation: Day Thirty-three

November 19, 2003

Today we got up at 7:30 AM, our regular time. We took a shower, got dressed and had our breakfast. We had to be at the Doctor's office [Doctor Griffis] for Joan's last radiation treatment at 12:00 PM. We arrived at 11:45 AM as usual and they took Joan right away as they always do. We brought some cookies for all including the other patients to have with the great coffee that is always there. Joan graduates today! That is what they call it when you finish your last session. Joan handled the radiation program like a real trooper. She did not have any complaints about anything at all. The only side effects that Joan had, was extreme tiredness and some redness on her chest which was over the operation area and under her arm where they took out the nodes. Joan did have some emotional days which could have come from being so tired and from just thinking about what she has been going through. I'm sure, in time, this will pass and, as we said before, everything is going to be OK. We now, or in a few weeks, after seeing all the Doctor's again, will be able to get on with our lives and be very grateful that Joan had the best Doctors and the best care from all of the Doctor's staff that you could get anywhere. In our hearts we know we could not have done any better. After Joan's radiation treatment, they made several appointments to see Doctor Iannotti on Monday November 24th 2003 at

2:00 PM at his Port St. Lucie office and to come back to see Doctor Griffis at the cancer center in Stuart on Dec. 18th at 10:00 AM. I'm sure these are follow up visits to see how Joan is doing and also to discuss what Joan will be going to do next. We believe all of the treatments are done, so I'm sure if there is anything else to do, it will be for us to do, like medicines and some kind of program for Joan to keep up with. We still have to see Doctor Vopal and find out about taking the port out. I'm also sure that there will be some kind of test to do to see if all is OK. We left the Doctor's office and came right home. Joan was very tired and so was I. I'm sure it is because we are wondering what is to take place next and when. For now we will just enjoy the next four days without any Doctor's appointments to go to. I thought we would get a break after the radiation program was over. Joan took a nap and I, you got it, did more paper work. I let Joan sleep most of the afternoon, or I should say until dinner was ready. I did not feel like cooking tonight so I went out for KFC. We like the chicken breast with the crunchy covering on it. We also like the coleslaw and the mashed potato with gravy. I like the potatoes and Joan likes the macaroni and cheese. We did not go there to have dinner, I brought it home. Joan was too tired to go out and the weather was kind of rainy. After we ate I had to make a few calls. I received a call from our daughter Doreen telling me that our oldest granddaughter Christy was hit by a car this morning while she was walking to her car in a parking lot. She was not hurt seriously, but was taken to the hospital by ambulance. She was badly bruised and had scrapes on her leg and ankle along with a painful back. She was very lucky. It could have been real bad. The doctor at the hospital said he did not think she should put any weight on her leg and ankle for at least three days. I called my daughter, Diane who is Christi's Mom and she said that she would be OK. I also talked to Christie and she did not sound too great to me. I guess she was quite shaken up. I thought about whether I should tell Joan tonight or wait until tomorrow when she was more awake. I could not wait until tomorrow because Joan was asking me what was going on and who called. Joan sensed that something was not right. I did tell Joan and of course she sort of went to pieces. After assuring Joan that Christie was really alright, she calmed down and was OK. I really think we have had it for today. I will say goodnight and will talk to you tomorrow. Goodnight.

November 20, 2003

Today we got up about 10:00 AM and of course the first thing on our mind was our granddaughter, Christie. We wondered how she did through the night. We did wait until after lunch to call. We called our daughter Doreen to see if she knew anything. We would have called Diane, our other daughter, and Christi's Mom, but we figured she would be very busy with taking care of Christie. Doreen said that Diane took Christie to her regular doctor for a follow up on what the hospital doctors did and that we should call Diane later in the day. I called Diane later and she said Christie was doing as well as could be expected. She did not have a good night but seemed to be OK now. The regular doctor said that Christie really got banged up and would most likely be laid up for a while. We will know more after a few days. Having our grandchild hurt kind of got our thoughts off what was going on with us. I really don't think this is what we needed. It would have been nicer if our minds were diverted by something happy going on. Joan is feeling good today, health wise. We are not doing anything but relaxing and trying to think about what we might do that would be fun. I'm sure we will come up with something. The rest of today will be spent taking it easy and checking on our Granddaughter. I will talk to you tomorrow. Goodnight.

November 21, 2003

We got up at 7:30 AM. We had to go to our regular doctor, Doctor Pinto for a fasting blood test, to check our cholesterol. We had this appointment for awhile, but forgot we had it until they called us yesterday to confirm it. We spent about two hours with the Doctor so we could bring him up to date on what has been going on with Joan. The appointment was for the both of us, but we thought it was best we bring him up to date on Joan's situation. It was a long appointment but very important that Doctor Pinto knew everything. After we left Doctor Pinto's office we were kind of hungry since we had not eaten since last night. We went to Perkins for breakfast. I like to go to Perkins. They have good pancakes and fix eggs any way you want them. After breakfast we went to Circuit City to get some things for my computer, we than went home. Joan was very tired and so was I. We were supposed to be on vacation and we haven't relaxed yet. Oh well, maybe we can start tomorrow. After we got home we did not do anything, but rest, Joan took a nap and I just laid on the coach and read until my eyes sort of closed. After we woke up it was time to start dinner. I am making dinner tonight. It will be spaghetti with meat sauce, salad and some nice French bread. It was pretty good. Am I a cook or what? I guess mostly or what. I think we will do our regular activities for tonight, T/V and go to bed. Goodnight.

Voice of the Children

If someone is in a similar situation what would your advise be to them?

My advice would be to show as much support and love as you can. I really feel that having a supportive and loving family makes all the difference in the world. Even though we could not be there every day I feel our love and strong desire for mom to get better helped her to be strong. *Diane*

Every situation is different but my advise to families that go thru this would be to just give a helping hand when ever possible, show support by showing your love and just being there whether it be a phone call to listen or just stopping by for a hug. *Kim*

I would advise them to make sure they find the right medical specialists to take care of business. Bedside manner is just as important as skill and reputation. My mother-in-law's cancer specialist was nationally renowned and yet he treated her as a specimen, not a person. I think a positive emotional outlook helps the recovery process. That's also why I think reading up on the experiences of others in the same situation helps you understand what to expect. I think that's why books like my father's are so important to have available. Ken

Family is such an important support system. We all need help a tone point in our lives and who better than our family to give it. I know that this is not always the case in some families. In times like this, we all need to find the strength to pull together and help in the fight giving the encouraging words show the love and affection that is needed to heal. We all pulled together. *Doreen*

November 22, 2003 On Vacation

November 23, 2003 On Vacation

November 24, 2003

The past two days were fantastic. We did absolutely what ever we wanted to do - no Doctors, no traveling and no appointments to keep. We slept until we woke up. We ate whenever we wanted and what ever we wanted. We did not think of anything related to any kind of a problem at all, except for our granddaughter who had been hit by a car. I really meant it, when I said we went on vacation. Christie, our granddaughter is now recuperating and will be OK. Today we had to get up early, or I should say I had to get up early. The electrician is coming to fix a couple of problems at 8:30 AM and I had better be up to great them. The electricians were working and I made breakfast for Joan and myself. After breakfast we did a few things around the house while we were waiting to leave for Joan's appointment with Doctor Iannotti. This is rather an important appointment, he is going to go over everything to date that has been going on with Joan. He, I assume, will tell us what is going to be next for Joan to do. We left for Doctor Iannotti's office at 1:15 PM and arrived at his office at 1:45 PM. This is the first time we had an appointment in his Port St. Lucie office. Doctor Iannotti has three offices that he works from, Port St. Lucie, Fort Pierce and Stuart. Each office is very nice and the staff at each office is also very nice. Some of the staff must travel to each of the offices. Doctor Iannotti examined Joan and said everything looked real good, I think he was happy that Joan did not get too much redness on her skin from the radiation. He told us that he would not have to see Joan for three months. Doctor Iannotti prescribed medicine for Joan to take to prevent the cancer from coming back. YES, Joan is now cancer free, and if she continues with the medicine and the check ups she should always be cancer FREE. This is the news that we wanted to hear, and you can be real sure that whatever program Joan must stay on to keep her CANCER FREE we will be doing. We will be going to Doctor Griffis on the 18th of December for a follow up visit. Doctor Iannotti thinks he will order a mammogram at that time which when taken will be sent to Doctor Vopal for him to check out. Doctor Griffis will also give us a follow up visit schedule for Joan to come and see him. I'm sure that when we see Doctor Vopal he will set up a follow up program for Joan. As time goes by I'm sure the follow up visits will get further apart. Doctor Iannotti could not have made Joan and I any happier than we are right now. We have been thinking about this moment for a long time. Being told that Joan is now cancer free is like telling a child they can have anything they want while in a toy store. We are too tired to do a dance or jump up and down with joy, but given a little time, LOOK OUT. For now I'm sure there will be a few tears of happiness and a lot of thank you to all that were so concerned about Joan. After we left Doctor Iannotti's office we went right home. I don't know if we were just tired or whether we just wanted to lie down next to each other and just think about what has happened to us and how happy we are about the outcome. We thought and talked for about two hours and were very content just being together with our thoughts of how fortunate we were to have things turn out the way they did. We had the very best of care along with the many prayers and love bestowed on us. I think we will have something to eat and watch some T/V until bed time. I think it is time to say goodnight. Talk to you tomorrow. Goodnight.

November 25 & 26, 2003

Tuesday - Today I believe will be a great day. The news we got yesterday will sink in even more as the next few days go by. Unlike so many days before today, we do not have to think about what Doctor or what procedure Joan has to see or do. There are a few things that have to be done, such as the follow up visits with Doctor Griffis and Doctor Vopal. Joan also will have to have a Mammogram, some more blood tests and the port will have to be removed. These are things that need to be done to close out the programs that Joan was on to cure her cancer problem. We will look forward to doing these few things so we can get back to a normal life, with all our friends and loved ones.

Wednesday – Today we thought a lot about our family and friends. We wanted to tell everyone, so we did a lot of talking on the phone, just letting them know as to what the outcome was with the visit Joan had with Doctor Iannotti. Of course everyone was very happy for Joan and me, and wished us all the best for the future. We are very lucky to have so many friends and loved ones. I think we would be lost were it not for all of you. We thank you all for your Love and thoughtfulness that you have given us. We especially want to thank every one for the many, many, prayers that were said for Joan to get well. Joan and I are looking forward to tomorrow, Thanksgiving day. We are spending Thanksgiving day with our daughter Kim, our son-in-law John and our four grandchildren – Sammy – Justin – Amanda – and Sierra. The only thing that could make us any happier, would be to have all our other children, Diane, Doreen and Ken with there spouses, Pat, Tony and Stephen and all our other grandchildren, Kristie, Kerri, AJ, Christopher, Jeff, Ryan, Dana, James and Christian,[WOW WHAT A FAMILY] with us also. I am sure they will be with us in our hearts and us with them in there hearts. We are two very lucky people. We will be going to our Son-in-law's Aunt and Uncle's house in Vero Beach, Florida. Irene and Lars have been very thoughtful of Joan and me and have invited us for the last three years to their house for Thanksgiving dinner. They are very delightful people and a pleasure to be with. We are really looking forward to tomorrow.

November 27, 2003 - Happy Thanksgiving

Today, as I told you we went to our son-in-law's Aunt and Uncle's house for Thanksgiving dinner. Vero Beach is about one hour North of Port St. Lucie. It was a very pleasant drive. They really had a full house, all of our son-in-law's family were there and a few more. I think there had to be at least thirty or more people. Of course our Daughter Kim and our four grand children being there made our day.

It was amazing to see how every thing was handled. There had to be enough food to feed at least twice the amount of people that were there. The food was wonderful and so was being with all the family and friends that were there. It was exactly what Joan and I needed. It was a perfect day. Joan did real good. She lasted from 3:00 PM to 8:30 PM before she needed to go home and lie down. I'd say for her first big outing in a long time, she did wonderfully. Joan did not start the medicine that Doctor Iannotti gave her on Monday. She was afraid that if she got any of the side effects, she might not have been able to go on Thanksgiving day and that would have been a shame. This is a Thanksgiving that Joan and I will always remember. We have so much to be thankful for and only hope that all that are in need of prayers will have the same results from there prayers that we received from all the prayers that were said for Joan. We love God and we know He loves us. That is all that any one really needs to know. Joan did take the medicine that Doctor Iannotti prescribed. This is the medicine that Joan will be taking for the next five years. The first prescription was on a trial basis to see if Joan could tolerate it. [It was at N/C] The second prescription if all goes well will be what Joan will be on for the five year program. Joan took the first pill on Thursday night at 11:00 PM and had a reaction on Friday morning after she was awake for a little while. The reaction was light headedness, which they said could happen. If it continues after a week or two Joan would have to tell Doctor Iannotti and he would have to change to another prescription. It is now Tuesday, six days after Joan took the first pill and it is starting to simmer down, so we are hoping it will work out OK with the pill she started with. This pill and all the follow up visits will be all we should have to do from now on. I think we are at the end of the cure for Joan's cancer problem. We just have to be very wary and very diligent on keeping up with the five year program and all the follow up visits. I can assure you that we will.

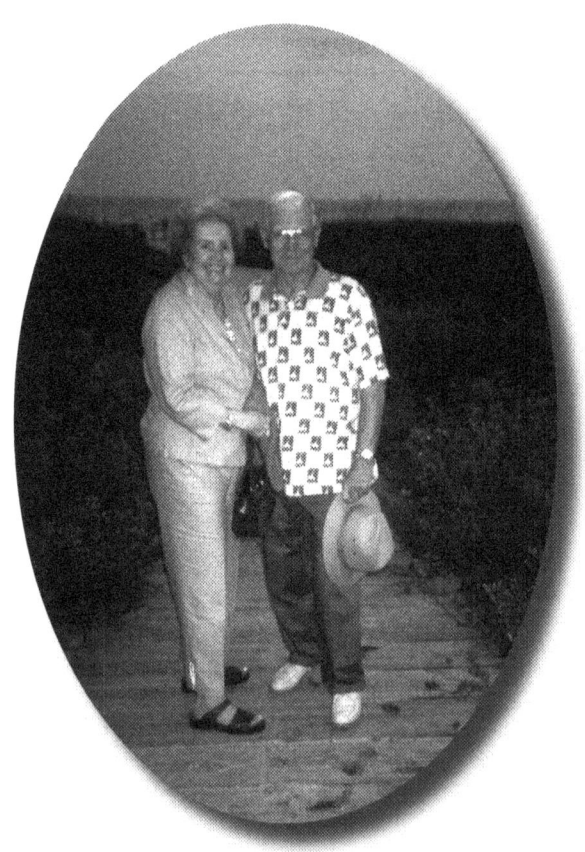

Happy Conclusion

*I*t has been about a month since I concluded my story about Joan's fight with breast cancer and how we handled it. The first couple of weeks did not change too much in the way Joan was feeling except for the emotional feelings for Joan and me. We both feel that we have been set free and could now start to get on with our lives.

After the first couple of weeks, Joan has been feeling a lot better. She no longer has any nausea and has much more energy to do some of the things she has wanted to do. She still gets tired very quickly, but that, I'm sure, will improve in time. As a matter of fact, Joan's beautiful head is now covered with hair—not much, but it's on its way.

We are both very thankful and feel that all the prayers said for my Joan have been answered. We are no looking forward to a happy future and again thank everyone for the support, prayers and love that you have given to Joan, to me and to our family.

I pray from the bottom of my heart that if you have been diagnosed with cancer or just know someone who has been diagnosed with cancer, that my story about how Joan and our family went through the treatments will be so some value to you and your loved ones.

The most important thing that I hope you get from my story is to make sure you always stay positive. Just keep thinking about the day your doctor will say to you that **You Are Now Cancer Free**.

The journey will be difficult at times, but there will also be good things that happen on the way to assure you that everything will turn out OK.

We said a lot of prayers, not only for ourselves but for all that might be in the same situation. All of our prayers and all the prayers from everyone else gave us the courage to always stay positive. Please know that we never stop praying for all who need prayers.

I could not be any happier that my story is over, that means that my Joan is al better and I no longer have a story to write about her.

I am also going to miss writing this story, because it brought me through some very upsetting moments when Joan was not feeling herself. I met some very lovely people through writing this story.

If I can be of any help, or if you want to ask me anything about what my story was all about, please feel free to get in touch with me. Just remember to stay positive and all will be well.

A Different Perspective

I can see how reading my father's book can help someone who has been diagnosed and doesn't quite know what to expect. I think emotions play a big part in the recovery process. For me though, reading my fathers book did something different. For the first 18 years of my life I was intimately involved with my parents and sisters everyday life as they were in mine. As I grew up and went away to college, got married, relocated and had a family of my own, the time I was able to spend with my parents and the involvement in each others lives became less and less. Now we only see each other a couple times a year, if that, and we talk once a week over the phone. I miss not being involved at all in my parents' and sisters' lives. As I was reading my dad's book a warm feeling came over me, and I felt that I was living with them once again and was intimately involved in their every day life for that year. I know it was a very hard year for them and I wish I could have really been there with them. I want to thank my mother for being strong enough to survive this horrible disease and I want to thank my dad, first, for taking such good care of my mom and second for taking the time to document every day of that year so other people can benefit from their experience and so I was able to intimately experience what they went through.

Ken Dickson, Jr.

Acknowledgements

Our ordeal started in March of 2003 and lasted until December 2003. Our goal was to make Joan cancer-free. I believe if we did not have three of the most fantastic doctors and all of their staff and technicians—I might not be writing this page at this time, if at all.

We cannot even begin to thank these doctors:

Doctor Vopal—Joan's breast doctor for cancer and surgery.

Doctor Iannotti—Joan's doctor for chemotherapy; Martin Memorial Center.

Doctor G.K. Griffis—Joan's doctor for her radiation treatment; Martin Memorial Cancer Center.

We also need to thank the many friends and loved ones who were so very supportive through Joan's whole ordeal. They never stopped praying and never stopped writing and calling. Whether they know it or not, their caring is what got us through this very difficult time. We are grateful for them and we love them from the bottom of our hearts

www.ingramcontent.com/pod-product-compliance
Lightning Source LLC
Chambersburg PA
CBHW051432280526
45785CB00003B/1259